Preface to the fourth edition

I have been greatly encouraged by the reception of the third edition, including Chinese and Arabic translations. I have taken the greatest care to make this new edition as up to date as possible, keeping the basic concepts clear as well as scientifically rigorous.

Like its predecessors, this edition is intended as an introduction to the science of medicinal chemicals – pharmacology – for nursing, medical and pharmacy students. Feedback from previous editions shows that nurse prescribers, doctors and pharmacists in mid-career have found it useful for updating their knowledge. *How Drugs Work* condenses only those aspects of pharmacology of direct relevance to everyday prescribing into a volume of 200 pages, without sacrificing accuracy, covering drug absorption, distribution, action, metabolism, excretion, adverse effects and interaction with other drugs.

Drug science continues its rapid advance, both in innovation (new drugs) and fundamental research (greater understanding of drug action). Two short chapters have been added – on the antidiabetic drugs, and on making a practice formulary – but every chapter has been revised.

As with previous editions, my aims remain:

1   To distil complex information into what is essential for the prescriber, without sacrificing scientific accuracy.
2   To convey to the newcomer with little or no prior knowledge my own enthusiasm for the intrinsically beautiful and important clinical science upon which 95% of medical treatment is based.
3   To provide readers with an understanding of how drugs work sufficient to make their prescribing and medication reviewing safer and more effective.

Your critical feedback will be welcomed!

Hugh McGavock
Cloughmills, Co. Antrim, UK
July 2015

For those who have fully mastered the contents of *How Drugs Work*, there is a companion volume, one level more advanced – *Pitfalls in Prescribing and How to Avoid Them* (2009). This will be of particular use to clinicians who are already prescribing, by reducing the risk of avoidable prescription-related illness.

Acknowledgements

I am indebted to many colleagues for advice, information and criticism, particularly to the staff of the Northern Ireland Regional Medicines and Poisons Information Service, for unfailing, rigorous and speedy responses to my many queries. I have had great support from my publishers over the past twelve years and wish to record my appreciation of their work.

Hugh McGavock
Cloughmills, Co. Antrim, UK
July 2015

Contents

To my dear wife, Betty,
and sons, James, Sam and Philip

1 Getting a drug into the body: absorption

It may seem a truism to state that unless a drug is absorbed into the body in sufficient amounts, it will not work.

However, prescribers are often unaware that the drug industry spends perhaps a quarter of its research budget for a new drug on pharmaceutics, i.e. devising the right presentation to ensure that the drug is effectively absorbed, properly distributed, and remains at its site of action long enough to produce an effect. This is often a major problem whose solution we clinicians take for granted, but it may have involved intense research activity and many millions of pounds of research investment.

Of course, this process is by no means a recent development. Over the past 45 years, the following advances have been made:

- capsules and enteric coatings (EC), which avoid, for example, degradation by gastric acid
- modified-release (MR) tablets, which extend the duration of action of the drug
- inactive pro-drugs, which the body's metabolic processes convert to active compounds
- skin patches for transdermal drug delivery
- subcutaneous implants for long-term treatment
- sophisticated inhalers
- drug-releasing vaginal rings and intrauterine devices (IUDs) as an effective means of long-term drug delivery in women
- dosage-adjustable self-injection devices, particularly for insulin-dependent diabetics.

Absorption processes

This chapter describes the five processes that feature in drug absorption:

- passive diffusion down a concentration gradient (most drugs)
- the cell membrane and fat-solubility of drugs (most drugs)
- active transport (some drugs)

- disintegration and dissolution of tablets (many drugs)
- presystemic metabolism (first-pass metabolism) (most drugs).

Passive diffusion down a concentration gradient

Only intravenous and inhaled anti-asthma drugs avoid the need for absorption across cell membranes. Most other drugs are absorbed from the intestine, skin or mucous membranes, mainly by passive diffusion across cell membranes from an area of high drug concentration to one of low concentration, until the concentrations in the two areas are in balance (equilibrium). They reach the blood capillaries by similar passive diffusion, and are distributed around the body.

The rate of absorption of a drug depends on three things: the concentration gradient, the surface area available for absorption and the fat-solubility of the drug itself.

The principle of the concentration gradient is the reason why oral drugs are best absorbed if given well before a meal, as this maximises their concentration in the small intestine, from which most oral drugs are absorbed. Note the very large surface area of the jejunal villi, which makes the jejunum an ideal site for the absorption of the majority of drugs.

The cell membrane and fat-solubility of drugs

Although the cells lining many blood capillaries, particularly the kidney glomerulus, have pores between them allowing relatively free passage of drug molecules, most other tissues, including the intestine, have few intercellular pores large enough to permit drug absorption.

To be absorbed, oral drugs must therefore cross the cell membranes of the intestinal villi. As in all cells, the membrane is composed of a double 'fatty' layer of phospholipid, arranged like a palisade (*see* Figure 1.1). Although this is a pictorial representation, it is close to the molecular reality revealed by the electron microscope. In essence, it means that there is a well-sealed fatty barrier between the intracellular and extracellular fluids.

Fat-soluble molecules, including some drugs, can pass directly through the cell membrane. But on the right of Figure 1.1, you see that ionised and water-soluble molecules and ions, including some drugs, cannot cross the cell membrane.

Without the innate property of phospholipids to form such membranes, cell life would be impossible, since cellular metabolism depends to a very large extent on the maintenance of strict intracellular control of water and ions such as sodium, potassium and calcium, chloride and bicarbonate, which require active transport into and out of the cell.

An excellent example of passive diffusion and fat solubility is the almost instantaneous absorption of the anti-anginal drug glyceryl trinitrate (GTN) across the buccal (mouth) mucosa. A GTN spray delivers a high concentration of this very lipid-soluble compound of very low molecular weight, which is absorbed almost as fast as an intravenous injection.

Drugs are usually formulated to make them as lipid-soluble as possible, and the pharmaceutical industry has produced a variety of chemical means of achieving this end.

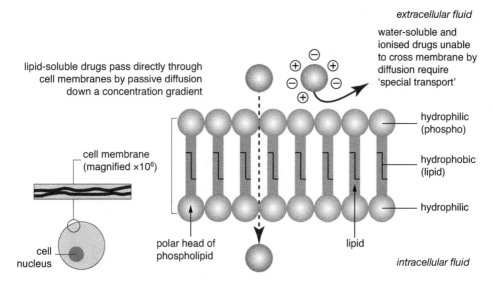

Figure 1.1 How drugs cross the cell membrane.

However, sometimes a drug's low lipid solubility is used to good effect, for example, with the use of aminosalicylates like mesalazine in the treatment of ulcerative colitis, and the antibiotics vancomycin and neomycin. In these examples, the aim is to get the drug into the lumen of the colon for therapeutic purposes, while avoiding systemic absorption.

Many drugs are weak acids or bases (in ionic equilibrium, part ionised, part un-ionised). In such cases, only the un-ionised form is sufficiently lipid-soluble to diffuse across phospholipid membranes.

Active transport across the intestinal mucosa

All cells have active transport mechanisms. These are essential for carrying ions, most sugars, and the amino acids into and out of the cell in a highly regulated fashion, which will be described later (*see* Chapter 9).

Active transport is not a very important means of drug absorption, although iron salts, levodopa for Parkinson's disease, the antithyroid drug propylthiouracil and the anticancer drug fluorouracil are actively transported across the intestinal mucosa.

However, it is important to realise at this stage that active transport exists, if only because many of our most effective renal, gastric and other drugs act by increasing or decreasing such cellular transport mechanisms. This is what happens every time we prescribe a proton pump inhibitor, for example to suppress the synthesis of gastric acid.

The importance of disintegration and dissolution of tablets in the stomach

Plain tablets first disintegrate and then dissolve in the stomach. Figure 1.2 shows the way in which a meal delays gastric emptying and, consequently, delays the absorption of any drug taken during or after food, and the effect that this may have on drug plasma concentration. So, to achieve maximal concentration in the small intestine, where most drugs are absorbed, a drug should be taken before food. This is a simple principle about which we sometimes need reminding, particularly when prescribing most antibiotics, where achieving an adequate tissue concentration is always paramount.

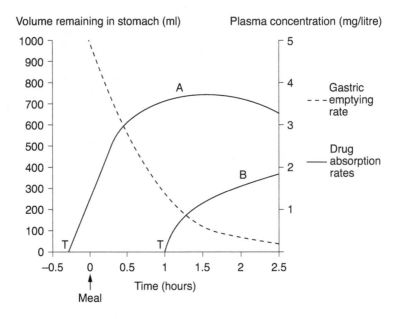

Figure 1.2 A tablet taken before a meal will dissolve in the stomach and enter the small intestine within 15 minutes (curve A); taken during or after a meal, the drug may not reach the intestine for 1–2 hours (curve B). T, time at which tablet is swallowed.

In contrast, where peak plasma concentrations may be associated with side-effects, drugs can be given with food to reduce peaks.

Many modern drugs are formulated to avoid early release; for example, an enteric coating is applied to the tablet when a drug is irritant to the gastric mucosa or when it is rendered inactive by gastric acid.

Modified-release (MR or LA) drugs are used when the duration of action of a short-acting drug needs to be prolonged, as with the heart drug nifedipine. These formulations may also be used when a gradual rise in plasma concentration is desirable, or for patient convenience, in the hope of improving compliance, if the patient has to take the drug less often.

It is essential to remember that when a branded MR product is selected for long-term therapy, as in the treatment of hypertension for example, that that branded version should always be repeated, because different MR brands of the same drug may have clinically important variations in absorption and plasma concentration. The ten MR nifedipine preparations cited in the *British National Formulary* (*BNF*) are a good example of this, in treating hypertension.

Among the commonest of self-medications are the antacids. If an antacid is consumed at the same time as certain oral drugs, a chemical reaction occurs between the drug and the antacid, rendering the drug ineffective and leading to treatment failure. This problem is considered in detail in Chapter 26.

Presystemic metabolism

Presystemic metabolism (breakdown of a proportion of a drug by specialised cellular enzymes) takes place before the drug reaches the systemic circulation. It occurs mainly in the liver, but a degree of breakdown also occurs in the intestinal mucosa (see below), lungs and skeletal muscle (*see* Figure 1.3).

Clearly, extensive metabolism results in a greatly decreased plasma concentration of drug. For example, only one-twentieth of the dose of levodopa survives first-pass metabolism in the liver, and a similar story exists for many drugs.

Practitioners rarely have to consider this factor, since drug dosage is designed to take into account such wastage. This explains the practical importance of bioavailability, which is the fraction of an oral dose that reaches the systemic circulation. Chapters 3 and 4 describe the chemical processes involved in drug metabolism.

Inactivation of drugs in the mucous membrane of the small intestine

The absorbing surface of the small intestine has a mechanism to detoxify toxins in food. As might be expected, the body treats most drugs as toxins, and a proportion of many commonly used drugs is inactivated in the intestinal villi, before absorption can occur. This mechanism will be described in Chapters 3 and 26.

Why does drug absorption matter to the prescriber?

Prescribers have to make decisions based on drug absorption every day. In the emergency situation, where the highest possible plasma concentration of a drug is required immediately, the drug is given intravenously, for example, intravenous furosemide (frusemide) for acute pulmonary oedema.

Intravenous injection can be difficult, for example in the treatment of an epileptic fit, when rectal administration of the highly lipid-soluble drug diazepam is the preferred and very effective route, as the rectum has an excellent blood supply. *See* A and B routes in Figure 1.3.

Inhalers and nebulisers are used to deliver anti-asthmatic beta$_2$-agonists and corticosteroids directly to the bronchioles and lung alveoli.

Skin conditions are usually treated by direct dermal application and the transdermal route is often used for hormone replacement therapy, and for relief of severe pain without regular injections.

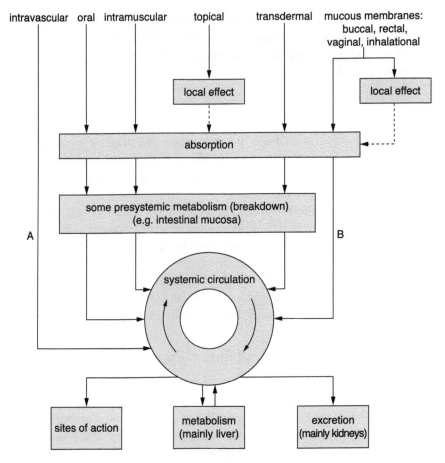

Figure 1.3 Choosing the appropriate route of drug administration.[2] Presystemic metabolism occurs in the intestinal mucosa, liver, lungs and skeletal muscle. A is the preferred route for most emergency drug administration, with B as a good alternative for some drugs, e.g. anti-epileptics, anti-asthmatics, anti-anginals (GTN), where rapid action is needed. The pecked arrow below 'local effect' shows that a proportion of many topical applications (e.g. skin, eye, vagina) is absorbed systemically.

Figure 1.4 shows the principle of the matrix-type skin patch.[1] All of the drugs derived from the cholesterol stem, including the male and female sex hormones and cortisol itself, are highly lipid-soluble and readily absorbed through the skin, as is fentanyl (Durogesic), the useful strong analgesic skin patch, for managing severe chronic pain.

It is sometimes forgotten to what extent potent synthetic steroids are absorbed systemically from dermal creams, and it is important to emphasise the quantity that should be applied, for example, 'finger-tip units' – *see* Figure 1.3 again.

On the other hand, drugs that are relatively lipid-insoluble, such as the antirheumatic non-steroidal anti-inflammatory drugs (NSAIDs), are poorly absorbed through the skin, and are not a logical way of achieving therapeutic concentrations of anti-inflammatory agents.

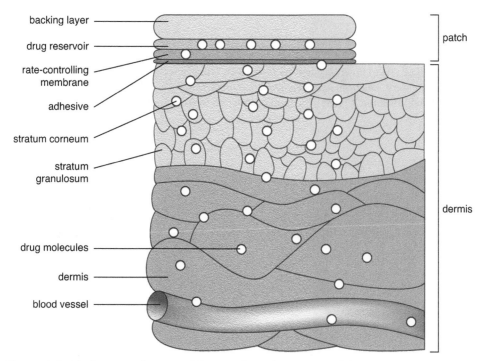

Figure 1.4 Mechanism of action of the transdermal matrix patch.[1]

Figure 1.3 summarises the routes of drug administration available to the prescriber. Which rate should be selected depends on the diagnosis, the urgency, the characteristics of the drug to be given, patient preference, and the need to avoid first-pass metabolism.

Key points

■ The main principles of drug absorption are:
  ● the disintegration and dissolution of tablets
  ● passive diffusion down a concentration gradient
  ● the cell membrane and fat-solubility of drugs
  ● active transport of ions and water-soluble drugs
  ● presystemic metabolism.
■ Drug formulations affect absorption.
■ The prescriber's aim should be the optimal drug-delivery route, i.e. the most appropriate and cost-effective.

References

1 Nachtigall LE (1995) Emerging delivery systems for estrogen replacement: aspects of transdermal and oral delivery. *American Journal of Obstetrics and Gynecology.* **173**: 993–7.
2 Kruk Z and Whelpton R (1985) Focus on drug action (series). *Mims Magazine.* **January**: 44.

2 Getting a drug to its site of action: distribution

In the first chapter, we considered the principles of drug absorption from the intestine and mucous membranes, the skin and the lungs into the bloodstream. The next stage in understanding drug action is to study the distribution of the absorbed drug by the blood circulating around the body, because unless a drug reaches its site of action in an adequate concentration, it will obviously not work.

Transport of drugs in the bloodstream

The rate at which a drug reaches any given part of the body and the amount of drug delivered depend entirely on the rate and volume of blood perfusing that part of the anatomy (*see* Figure 2.1).

In well-perfused tissues, such as the brain, heart, kidneys and lungs (Curve 2), the concentration of drug following a bolus (rapid) intravenous injection quickly reaches a maximum which is higher than that achieved in any other tissue. Tissues in the well-perfused group will therefore achieve effective plasma concentrations relatively easily and quickly.

In tissues with intermediate rates of blood perfusion, the maximum drug concentration is lower than that in Curve 2, and is reached considerably later (Curve 3). In tissues with poor blood perfusion, such as fat, there is a prolonged delay in reaching the maximum drug concentration (Curve 4), which is lower than that in the better-perfused tissues.

Figure 2.1 represents plasma and tissue drug concentrations following intravenous injection, which is the optimal drug delivery route in terms of achieving maximal tissue concentration without first-pass metabolism. The normal route in most therapies is, of course, the oral route, in which bioavailability, i.e. the proportion of drug actually reaching the systemic circulation, is commonly reduced by incomplete intestinal absorption and first-pass metabolism in the liver.

It may be of interest to note that bioavailability is calculated by comparing the area under curve (AUC) for Curve 1, resulting from the intravenous injection of a drug, with the AUC resulting from an identical oral dose.

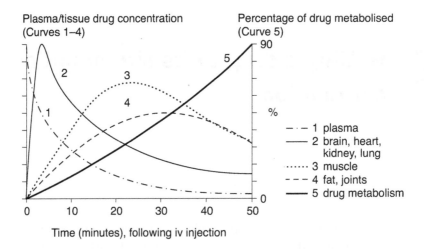

Figure 2.1 Plasma and tissue concentrations of a fat-soluble drug following bolus intravenous injection, and percentage of drug metabolised.

What happens next?

The value of Figure 2.1 is that it provides a mental picture of the entire time course of drug action. Having described the maximum concentrations in different tissues, let us follow the curves along the time axis.

Following Curve 1, why does the plasma concentration of a drug fall off so quickly? This happens for two reasons. The first is that under a positive concentration gradient, the drug passes out of the capillaries into the interstitial fluid bathing the body cells until there is equilibrium between the plasma and interstitial fluid concentrations. In the interstitial fluid, the drug has access to the tissue cell receptors upon which it will exert its therapeutic effect (there is more about this topic in Chapters 6–10).

The second reason for the rapid fall in plasma concentration seen in Curve 1 (and for the progressively slower fall of tissue concentration seen in Curves 2, 3 and 4) is that on every circulation of blood through the liver, a proportion of most drugs is metabolised and usually rendered inactive. We shall consider drug metabolism and excretion in the next two chapters.

Continuing our study of Figure 2.1: how does the drug concentration in the tissues fall? Well, it is simply due to a reversal of the concentration gradient. As the plasma concentration (*see* Curve 1) falls due to drug metabolism (*see* Curve 5), so the concentration in the tissues comes to exceed that in the bloodstream, and the drug diffuses from the tissues back into the capillaries.

The last thing to note in Figure 2.1 is that, although the peak tissue drug concentration is lower in Curves 3 and 4, the drug remains in these tissues much longer. Likewise, the time taken for the tissue drug concentration to fall to half its original peak concentration (its half-life or $t_{1/2}$) is longer in Curve 3 than Curve 2, and longest of all in Curve 4.

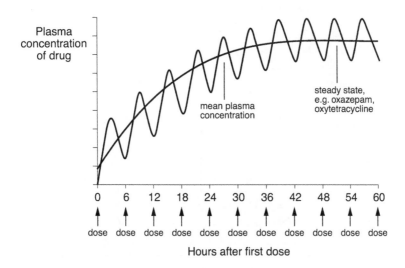

Figure 2.2 Plasma concentration of a drug with a half-life of nine hours after six-hourly oral doses – the 'steady state' concept.

'Steady state'

If a suitable dosage interval is chosen, the first six or seven doses will be absorbed before the preceding doses have been fully eliminated, i.e. there will be a progressive accumulation of drug in the plasma and tissues, as shown in Figure 2.2. So, for many drugs, a 'steady state' of plasma and tissue concentration is reached, typically after six or seven oral doses.

At steady state, the drug concentration in all tissues is relatively constant (input balancing output), as opposed to the scenario shown in Figure 2.1. This is why good patient compliance (adherence) with dosage schedules is important to achieve maximal therapeutic results (efficacy) – *see* Chapter 30.

However, drugs like amoxycillin ($t_{\frac{1}{2}}$ 1.5 hours) never reach steady state with normal 6-hourly oral dosing, and good compliance is even more vital.

Protein binding – does it matter?

When protein bound, drugs are largely inactive. Many drugs bind loosely to plasma albumin and other proteins, but are rapidly released as free drug when their plasma concentration falls (*see* Figure 2.3).

Protein binding is only a problem when one drug, such as the heart drug verapamil, displaces another, such as digoxin, from its binding site, leading to a sudden release of free, unbound drug and possible toxicity. There are few such examples.

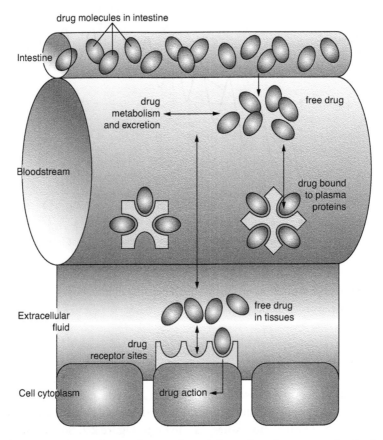

Figure 2.3 A proportion of many drugs is loosely bound to plasma proteins in the bloodstream. However, this does not have a prolonged effect on the plasma concentration or drug action, as the molecules are readily released when the free drug concentration falls. Examples of drugs that are largely protein bound are: diazepam, ibuprofen, propranolol, flucloxacillin, erythromycin, phenytoin, nifedipine and verapamil. (*Figure is not to scale.*)

Warfarin is 99% bound to plasma proteins, and is displaced by a number of drugs. Appendix 1 of the *British National Formulary* (*BNF*) should be consulted whenever any drug is co-prescribed with warfarin.

Hydrophilic drugs

The distribution of fat-soluble (lipophilic) drugs has been described. Water-soluble (hydrophilic) drugs are mainly partially ionised – weak acids or bases have different kinetics (their absorption, distribution, metabolism and excretion):

- they are slowly and only partially absorbed

- they are not subject to significant first-pass metabolism in the liver
- they do not cross the healthy blood–brain barrier
- they are only slightly protein-bound, or not protein-bound at all
- they are filtered unchanged by the kidney, without reabsorption (*see* Chapter 4 on drug excretion). Examples of such hydrophilic drugs are the antibiotic phenoxymethylpenicillin and the heart drugs lisinopril and atenolol.

The drug industry can often modify hydrophilic and/or ionised drug molecules so as to render them partially lipophilic.

Key points

- Distribution of a drug around the body is not uniform.
- Well-perfused tissues receive higher drug concentrations, faster.
- With good compliance (adherence) by patients, many drugs used for long-term maintenance therapy reach 'steady state', in which all body tissues receive a similar drug concentration.
- Protein binding of drugs is usually not important and does not affect efficacy.
- The main differences in the body's handling of hydrophilic drugs are summarised.

3 Inactivating drugs: phase 1 drug metabolism

One of the main reasons that we can use drugs as therapy, without poisoning the patient, is that the body is generally very good at inactivating and getting rid of them – metabolism and excretion.

In Chapter 1, we saw that the majority of effective drugs are relatively fat-soluble, since these pass easily across cell membranes during absorption from the intestinal villi and distribution around the body. In Chapter 2, we saw that the more fat-soluble drugs escape more easily from the peripheral capillaries into the interstitial fluid bathing the body cells.

Why bring up fat-solubility again? Because the most effective way of making a drug inactive or less active is often to render it less fat-soluble and more water-soluble, which can be done in various ways, for example by adding an oxygen atom (oxidation), or adding an OH^- ion (hydroxylation) or by removing a CH_3 group (dealkylation). This is what happens in phase 1 metabolism in the liver. How this occurs is a most interesting topic that is vital to understanding the clinical problem of drug interaction, which is the cause of a significant proportion of prescription-related illness. Many of these adverse drug events could be avoided if all prescribers had a clear grasp of the concepts in this chapter.

CYP isoenzymes (isoforms) – the P450 monooxygenase system

To understand hepatic drug metabolism is to go back several hundred million years to the original vertebrates – the fishes. In all natural environments, the food supply is contaminated to a greater or lesser extent. Ingestion of toxins from plants, rotting food, bacteria or fungi risks death from poisoning. Any animal species that can detoxify such toxins clearly has a greatly enhanced survival probability.

However, there are hundreds of environmental toxins that require many different enzymes in order to render them all inactive. Thus, during evolution vertebrates have developed an extensive battery of enzymes that render toxins inactive by reducing their fat-solubility (*see* Figure 3.1). This battery is the cytochrome P450 oxidase system, or CYP.

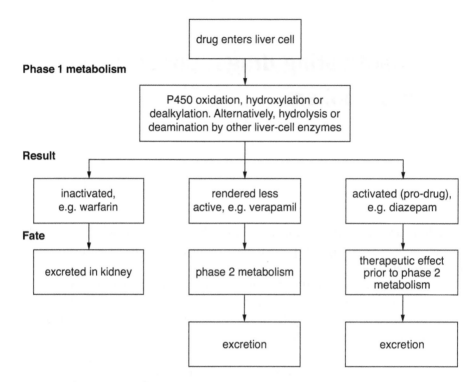

Figure 3.1 The concepts of phase 1 drug or toxin metabolism.

CYP comprises a wide range of isoenzymes (isoforms) of which one or more will be able to deactivate almost any given toxin, including most drugs. Figure 3.2 shows the catalytic reaction sequence of the CYP enzymes. Apart from hormones, all drugs are foreign substances (xenobiotics) and therefore potential toxins and they are treated as such by CYP in the liver. Those drugs or poisons that the CYP system cannot metabolise are processed by other enzyme systems, also in the liver.

Figure 3.2 shows that phase 1 drug metabolism is by no means difficult to understand. Figures 3.1 and 3.2 together explain the main concepts involved.

Most of the CYP enzymes involved in drug metabolism are in the liver, but some are found in the intestinal epithelium and the kidney also. They have been classified into 17 groups and many subgroups. Since their discovery 45 years ago, research has shown that they exist in many different isoforms (variations on a similar, iron-containing protein structure). It will probably be some decades before the complexity of the CYP system is fully understood. Table 3.1 gives some examples of CYP isoforms, with some of the drugs they metabolise. CYP groups 1–3 are involved in the majority of drug metabolism in man, particularly CYP3A4 and CYP3A5 (40% of all phase 1 reactions).

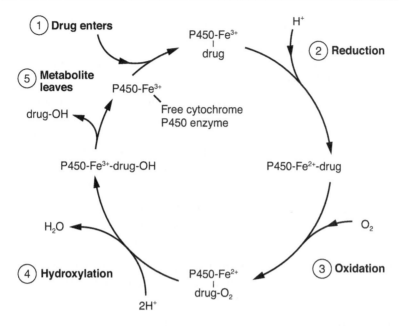

Figure 3.2 A scheme showing phase 1 hydroxylation by cytochrome P450 metabolism. The sequence of events should be read clockwise from 1 to 5. This is an enzymatic cycle in which, after the metabolite has left, the enzyme is regenerated to repeat the reaction cycle.

P450 inhibition and induction

The inactivation of fat-soluble drugs is largely dependent on hepatic (liver) metabolism, and anything that affects this will also affect the plasma concentration of drugs. Certain drugs disturb CYP function in one of two different, and opposite, ways: drugs may reduce CYP enzyme action (inhibition) or enhance enzyme action (induction). These effects become important when two drugs are co-prescribed, one of which inhibits or induces the CYP on which the other is dependent for its metabolism. As CYP enzymes metabolise drugs, it follows that inhibition of CYP will slow the second drug's metabolism and so lead to an increase in its plasma concentration, possibly to toxic levels. Induction of CYP, on the other hand, will speed up the second drug's metabolism and cause a reduction in its plasma concentration and potential treatment failure. Dozens of drugs are affected by these processes, and Tables 3.2 and 3.3 summarise those of greatest importance.

As mentioned in Chapter 1, the epithelium of the small intestine has a copious supply of metabolic enzymes, particularly CYP3A4, whose function is the inactivation of toxins in food. This enzyme also inactivates a proportion of many drugs, but the standard dosage of these drugs is set to make allowance for this 'wastage'. Unfortunately, grapefruit, grapefruit juice and bitter (Seville) oranges block the intestinal CYP, allowing a greater proportion of many oral drugs to be absorbed, leading to excessive plasma drug concentrations. Chapter 26 considers this problem in detail. It would be a very useful hour-long exercise for readers to look up each of the drugs in the left column of Tables 3.2

Table 3.1 Some clinically-important cytochrome P450 isoforms, listed according to the proportion of drugs metabolised by each isoform.

CYP Isoform	% of drugs metabolised	Examples of commonly used drugs metabolised by this enzyme isoform
CYP3A4, 5, 7	40%	Some macrolide antibiotics (e.g. erythromycin), many calcium-channel blockers (e.g. nifedipine), some benzodiazepines (e.g. triazolam), some statins (e.g. atorvastatin), some antivirals, some antihistamines, some immune modulators (anti-rejection drugs), some anti-arrhythmics, and many others
CYP2D6	20%	Several antipsychotics (e.g. haloperidol), many antidepressants (tricyclics and SSRIs), most beta-blockers, codeine and many others
CYP2C9	10%	Warfarin, phenytoin, most NSAIDs, several oral hypoglycaemics, some angiotensin II blockers and others
CYP2C19	10%	All proton pump inhibitors (e.g. omeprazole), indometacin, phenytoin, phenobarbital and others
CYP1A2	10%	Theophylline, caffeine, paracetamol, naproxen and others

Note. The CYP 'numeral/letter/numeral' is a biochemical classification. What matters in this table is that each individual CYP metabolises specific drugs. Some drugs can be metabolised by more than one CYP isoform, though one isoform usually predominates.

and 3.3 in Appendix 1 of the *British National Formulary* (*BNF*).* This will convince you of the importance to patient safety of understanding enzyme inhibition and induction. It will also show you that the best way to cope with this prescribing responsibility is to use a primary care computer software package like EMIS, which will 'flag up' dangerous drug:drug interactions in a few seconds, for the individual patient. And even if your computer has 'crashed', you will know where to seek the information in the *BNF*! Most pharmacies in the UK and Ireland screen prescriptions using First Databank drug interaction software (GB), or ALCHEMIST 3000 or MPS (Ireland). These tables include many of our most commonly used primary care drugs. However, it would do no harm to have a checklist on your desk, such as these tables, to refer to every time one of the drugs in the left-hand column is co-prescribed with another drug. A warning sticker on A4 record folders or a 'stop and check' signal on the computer record would help to prevent the harm that often occurs due to one drug's inhibition or induction of a second drug's metabolism.

Enzyme induction and inhibition are only two of the different types of drug:drug interactions that are of clinical importance. We shall consider all of them in Chapter 26, where you will meet these tables again!

---

* *BNF = British National Formulary*

For the sake of completeness it is worth noting that, at therapeutic doses, there is more than enough of the specific P450 enzyme available to metabolise most drugs rapidly, i.e. the metabolic processes are rarely saturated except in poisonous dosages.

Table 3.2 Drugs which *inhibit* the P450 enzymes which metabolise other drugs, thus increasing the plasma concentration of the latter drugs, possibly to toxic levels.

Drug group	*Main individual drugs in group and comments (italics)*
The imidazole anti-fungals (effective oral medication)	ketoconazole, fluconazole, itraconazole, miconazole. *Do not prescribe without checking BNF, Appendix 1, for interactions with existing medication*
Cimetidine, H_2 blocker (the original but now superseded gastric acid suppressant)	Dozens of serious interactions. **Do not prescribe.** *The other H_2 blockers are safer – ranitidine, famotidine and nizatidine*
Macrolide antibiotics (powerful broad-spectrum drugs)	erythromycin, clarithromycin. Dozens of serious interactions. *Do not prescribe without checking BNF, Appendix 1, for interactions with existing medication*
SSRI antidepressants (effective treatments, many side-effects, much overused)	fluoxetine, fluvoxamine, paroxetine, sertraline, citalopram. A score of serious interactions. *Do not prescribe without checking BNF, Appendix 1, for interactions with existing medication*
The effective, often used, anti-arrhythmic amiodarone (many side-effects, needs constant monitoring – *see BNF 2.3.2*)	Interacts with warfarin (which often has to be co-prescribed) and ten other drugs, four of them heart drugs. *Be suspicious of all new symptoms occurring in patients taking amiodarone and seek specialist help*
The proton pump inhibitors (very effective acid-suppressants, much overused, many side-effects)	omeprazole, esomeprazole, lansoprazole. Ten serious interactions. *Do not prescribe without checking BNF, Appendix 1, for interactions with existing medication*
The 4-quinolone antibiotics (powerful, overused, broad-spectrum drugs)	ciprofloxacin, norfloxacin, levofloxacin, ofloxacin, moxifloxacin. Interact with theophylline, methotrexate, coumarins, zolmitriptan and oestrogens. *Use only on certain diagnosis of bacterial infection and check BNF, Appendix 1*
The powerful anti-anaerobic antibiotic, metronidazole	Avoid use in patients taking phenytoin, barbiturates, primidone, fluorouracil, lithium or alcohol
The sulphonamides	Avoid use in patients taking phenytoin, coumarins, methotrexate and amiodarone (mechanism unclear)

(continued)

Drug group	Main individual drugs in group and comments (italics)
The anti-gout prophylactic allopurinol	Avoid use in patients taking ciclosporin, coumarins, the antiviral didanosine and theophylline. *The long-term management of gout should be under specialist supervision*
Two calcium-channel blockers (effective cardiac drugs)	verapamil and diltiazem. A dozen serious drug interactions. *Do not prescribe without checking BNF, Appendix 1, for interactions with existing medication*
Ethyl alcohol	Enhances the effect of many drugs, not necessarily via P450 inhibition. *See full page in BNF, Appendix 1. You will be amazed and enlightened!*
Grapefruit juice and grapefruit and bitter oranges	Enhances the effects of a score of drugs. *See BNF, Appendix 1. Patients on long-term medication should avoid it.*

Table 3.3 Important enzyme inducers. Drugs which *induce* the P450 enzymes which metabolise other drugs, and thus reduce the plasma concentration of the latter drugs, resulting in treatment failure.

Drug group	Main individual drugs in group and comments (italics)
All barbiturates and primidone	phenobarbital, amylobarbital, butobarbital, secobarbital, primidone. Over 20 serious interactions. *Specialist use only, but remember that the specialist may not know which other drugs the patient is taking. Do not prescribe without checking BNF, Appendix 1, for interactions with existing medication*
Two specialist anti-epileptics	phenytoin, carbamazepine. Over 20 serious interactions each. *The italics above apply. Note also that most anti-epileptics alter the plasma concentration of other anti-epileptics as well as unrelated drugs. See long BNF warning at start of Section 4.8.1. Combination therapy of epilepsy is sometimes unavoidable*
Anti-tuberculous drugs, the rifamycins	rifampicin, rifabutin. Over 40 serious interactions. *The italics above apply (specialist use). See long BNF cautions and guidance at start of Section 5.1.9, and full page of drug interactions in BNF Appendix 1*
St John's Wort – a very commonly used self-medication herbal remedy	Included in many impure, unstandardised herbal remedies, often sold in pharmacies! Over 20 serious interactions. *Make it your practice to ask all patients if they are taking herbals (they may not think of herbals as 'medicines').*

(continued)

Drug group	Main individual drugs in group and comments (italics)
St John's Wort (*cont.*)	*If they are using St John's Wort, check the full column of interactions in the BNF, Appendix 1, e.g. this herbal can cause failure of HIV treatment, and oral contraception failure* *As a general rule, patients should be warned to avoid all herbals if they are taking any prescription drug*
SSRI antidepressants (often unnecessary in mild depression)	fluoxetine, fluvoxamine, sertraline. A dozen serious interactions, particularly with antivirals and antipsychotics. *Check existing medication for SSRI interaction, using BNF, Appendix 1, before prescribing*
Two antivirals	efavirenz, nevirapine. Over ten serious interactions each. *Do not prescribe without checking BNF, Appendix 1 against existing medications*
One antifungal drug	griseofulvin, an older but still useful drug, sometimes used for several months. Interacts with several drugs, including oestrogens and progestogens (risk of contraceptive failure). *Study BNF, Appendix 1, before prescribing*

Drug interaction software packages, of which there are now several versions, should be used whenever there is the slightest doubt as to the compatibility of two or more co-prescribed drugs. Your UK Regional Medicines Information Service is only a phone call away (see inside front cover of your *BNF*). Its staff are the ultimate source of drug information for the prescriber. Your call will be logged and serve to indemnify you legally, should that become necessary.

Pharmacologically active phase 1 metabolites

It is also important to know that while phase 1 metabolism usually inactivates a drug or poison, in some cases the metabolite retains a pharmacological effect, although this is usually weaker than the effect of the parent drug.

In a few, but often fatal, cases the metabolite is highly toxic. Paraquat is one example of this – the metabolite releases a reactive oxygen species – and paracetamol overdose is another – the metabolite binds with liver cell macromolecules. Cell death is the result in both cases.

Conversely, quite a number of commonly prescribed drugs are pro-drugs, which are activated by phase 1 metabolism (*see* Figure 3.1). These include morphine, codeine, enalapril, amitriptyline and diazepam.

Alcohol and phenytoin

Alcohol, that ubiquitous social lubricant/drug/poison, is not metabolised by the P450 system, but by alcohol dehydrogenase and aldehyde dehydrogenase, which are also found in the liver.

The capacity of these two enzymes is limited, hence the slow metabolism of alcohol, leading to inebriation and sometimes loss of driving licence! 'Saturation' of the enzymes occurs on consumption of 1–2 units of ethanol, after which the ethanol concentration in the plasma, and consequently the breath, rises inexorably with successive drinks.

Saturation of the enzyme that processes the anti-epileptic phenytoin also occurs at the lower therapeutic dosages, after which its plasma concentration slowly reaches toxic levels. Prescribers need to be aware of the huge individual variability in phenytoin metabolic capacity, especially in children.

Other sites of drug metabolism

All body tissues have some metabolic activity. Those with medically significant metabolic capacity include the lungs, which metabolise most prostanoids (*see* Chapter 8), the kidneys, which metabolise serotonin and norepinephrine (noradrenaline), the intestine, which metabolises salbutamol, and plasma, which metabolises suxamethonium.

In every case, extrahepatic metabolism is due to the presence of the specific metabolic enzymes in the tissue involved.

Key points

- Phase 1 drug metabolism occurs mainly via the cytochrome P450 enzyme system (CYP).
- Metabolism occurs mainly in the liver, where P450 enzymes are concentrated.
- Phase 1 metabolism makes a drug more water soluble, less able to cross cell membranes and more easily excreted.
- The chemical reactions of phase 1 are oxidation, hydroxylation, dealkylation, reduction and hydrolysis.
- Pro-drugs are intentionally activated by phase 1 metabolism.
- Several common drugs either inhibit or induce the liver enzymes, which can lead to some of the most serious drug:drug interactions.

4 Phase 2 drug metabolism and methods of excretion

Chapters 1 and 2 described the processes and problems of getting drugs into the body and onwards to their sites of action. The processes of deactivating and eliminating drugs are also important for the prescriber, not to mention the patient! The drug that cannot be metabolised is a poison!

In Chapter 3 we looked at phase 1 of drug metabolism, which involves oxidation and hydroxylation reactions, among others, to inactivate the drug and render it more water-soluble.

The result of the first phase of drug metabolism is that the metabolite is more easily excreted via the kidneys, which are by far the most important route of drug excretion. Many drugs are excreted unchanged in the urine, and most of the rest are excreted as phase 1 or phase 2 metabolites.

Drugs that require further metabolism

The phase 1 metabolites of some important drugs are not water-soluble enough or polar enough for excretion, e.g. the metabolites of aspirin, morphine and methyldopa. These, and others, undergo further enzymatic chemical processing in the liver, known as phase 2 metabolism.

In this phase, the drug or its phase 1 metabolite is chemically bound (conjugated) to one of a number of chemical groups, including glucuronide, sulphate or acetyl groups, to create a larger, polarised molecule (*see* Figure 4.1).

The resulting conjugated drug is usually inactive pharmacologically, and very much more water-soluble and therefore more easily excreted in urine or bile. Surprisingly, some drugs are activated by conjugation – morphine-6-glucuronide is more active than morphine itself!

A number of the body's own products are conjugated before excretion, e.g. the steroid hormones and bilirubin. Neonatal jaundice is due to the relative inability of the newborn liver to conjugate excess bilirubin.

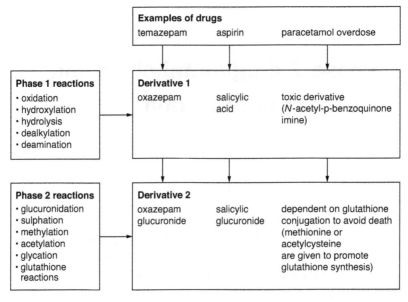

Figure 4.1 The reactions that can occur in phase 1 and 2 drug metabolism, and some examples of the products formed.

In some cases, drug metabolism produces a more active form of the drug than that taken orally – the jargon for this is the concept of the original as a 'pro-drug'. In a few cases, the metabolite is toxic. *See* Table 4.1.

Table 4.1 Some drugs that produce active or toxic metabolites.

Inactive (pro-drugs)	Active	Toxic
heroin codeine	morphine and morphine-6-glucuronide	
propranolol	4-hydroxypropranolol	
paracetamol		n-acetyl-p-benzo-quinone imine
imipramine	desmethylimipramine	
amitriptyline	nortriptyline	
diazepam	nordiazepam, oxazepam	
cortisone	hydrocortisone	
prednisone	prednisolone	
cyclophosphamide	phosphoramide mustard	
chloral hydrate	trichloroethanol	
azathioprine	mercaptopurine	
	sulphonamides	acetylated derivatives
enalapril	enalaprilat	
zidovudine	zidovudine triphosphate	

Excretion of drugs and their metabolites from the kidney

Figure 4.2 represents the function of a single renal tubule, as regards drug and metabolite excretion. Following through the numbering from left to right:

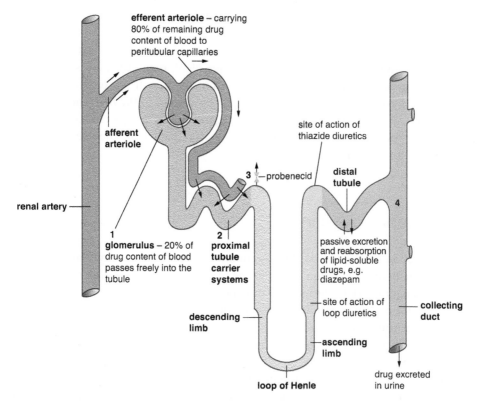

Figure 4.2 Processes involved in the renal excretion of drugs and drug metabolites; *see* text for further discussion. Arrows show drug/metabolite movement. *Not to scale.*

1 Approximately 20% of the drug content of blood perfusing the kidney will pass freely from the glomerulus into the renal tubule. The remaining 80% is carried in the efferent arteriole to the proximal convoluted tubule.

2 Two carrier systems in the tubular cells (one for acids, OAT,[*] the other for bases, OCT[†]) actively transport the drug metabolite from the capillary into the proximal tubule unidirectionally. Examples include: acetazolamide, aminosalicylate, furosemide (frusemide), indometacin, penicillins, thiazide diuretics, dopamine, morphine, quinine, serotonin, amiloride and triamterene.

---

[*] OAT = organic anion transporter
[†] OCT = organic cation transporter

3 Probenecid affects the transport of both penicillin and uric acid in opposite ways. It is used primarily to prolong the action of penicillin as it retards its excretion, but also in gout prophylaxis as it inhibits the reabsorption of uric acid. Sulfinpyrazone also inhibits the reabsorption of uric acid and is used in the treatment of gout.

4 Water is then reabsorbed in the collecting duct and the drug or drug metabolite is excreted in the urine.

5 Drugs which remain lipid-soluble are only slowly excreted by the kidney because they are reabsorbed into the renal tubular cells from the lumen.

The importance of renal excretion highlights the need to consider renal impairment when prescribing for elderly patients. By the age of 70, renal function is only 50% of its youthful maximum in most people. This means that the drug-excreting capacity is also reduced by around 50%. Hence the frequent warnings in the *BNF* and *MIMS* (the pharmaceutical industry's proprietary list) regarding the dosage reduction of many drugs when prescribing for elderly patients. (*See also* Chapter 24: The scientific basis of prescribing for the elderly.)

Enterohepatic cycling

Biliary excretion of drug metabolites is common, but results in only limited elimination from the body. The reason is that in the intestine, enzymes break the conjugation bond releasing free drug, a proportion of which is then reabsorbed into the circulation in its active form. Why mention biliary excretion at all, then? First, because it becomes an important route of excretion when renal function is poor. Second, because two commonly prescribed classes of drugs are affected – the benzodiazepines and the oral contraceptives.

Diazepam and its active metabolites are eventually conjugated as glucuronides in phase 2 reactions: *see* Figure 4.3 (1). A proportion of the diazepam glucuronide passes in the bile into the intestine (2). Intestinal enzymes split the glucuronide bond releasing free diazepam (3) which is then reabsorbed (4).

This process is called enterohepatic cycling, and is part of the reason for the very prolonged half-life of diazepam. Ultimately, most diazepam excretion occurs via the kidneys, slowly.

Enterohepatic cycling is also the reason why such low doses of oestrogen can be used in the contraceptive pill and patch. The oestrogen is repeatedly recycled (*see* Figure 4.3) and so maintains its anovulatory function.

Disruption of enterohepatic cycling explains why diarrhoea from any cause, including the therapeutic use of antibiotics, results in plasma concentrations of oestrogen inadequate to suppress ovulation. Women should be repeatedly reminded of the need to take additional precautions in such circumstances. Rapid diarrhoeal peristalsis greatly reduces the time available for enterohepatic recycling, leading to contraceptive failure, since more oestrogen is excreted.

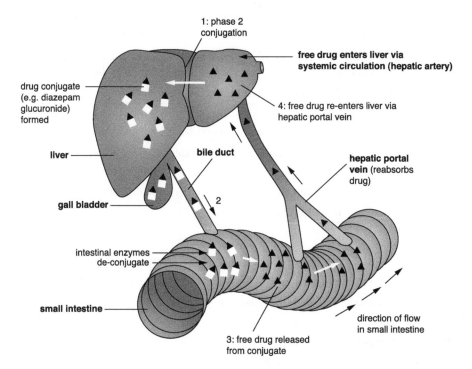

Figure 4.3 Enterohepatic cycling is important in the metabolism of some drugs; *see* text for further discussion.

Drugs in breast milk

Excretion of drugs in breast milk is not a maternally significant route of excretion, but may be very harmful to the breastfed baby.

Note that maternal consumption of many of these drugs may be unavoidable – hence the importance of the prescriber's awareness of potential harm to the infant.

Table 4.2 is a useful short guide for prescribers on this topic. It would do no harm to insert a copy in the clinical record of every breastfeeding mother as a checklist in case any prescription is needed, apart from those normally given postpartum (after birth). Table 4.2A includes most of the maternal drugs where breastfeeding is contraindicated. However, in many cases, breastfeeding may proceed with caution. Table 4.2B is to remind the prescriber to monitor the infant regularly, looking for signs of the stated effect. If in any doubt, seek specialist advice. Reference 1 is a useful source of guidance, updated every two years. A further problem caused by the excretion of drugs in milk is that antibiotics and other growth enhancers added to cattle feed may be excreted into cows' milk and can cause allergic responses in humans. If in doubt, seek expert advice. The *BNF* now gives no list of drugs to be avoided in the breastfeeding patient.

Table 4.2 Adverse effects of some *maternal* drugs on the breastfed baby;[2] this table is not comprehensive and prescribers should consult their Regional Medicines Information Service when prescribing for breastfeeding women.

A If the mother is taking the following drugs, the baby must NOT be breastfed:

Maternal drug	Effect on breastfed infant
antipsychotics	although secreted in small amounts in milk, animal studies indicate possible effects on the developing nervous system
antivirals	breastfeeding is contraindicated in mothers with AIDS/HIV infection
aspirin	risk of Reye's syndrome and hypoprothrombinaemia
cancer chemotherapy (cytotoxics)	toxic to infant's tissues
ciprofloxacin	reaches high concentrations in milk and will disrupt the baby's intestinal flora and cause other side-effects
immunosuppressive drugs	will harm the infant's immature immune system
SSRI antidepressants	best avoided
radiochemicals	radiation hazard
iodine	concentrates in milk, with risk of hypothyroidism and goitre
vigabatrin (antiepileptic)	possible effect on nervous system

B Breastfeeding may usually proceed (with caution) if the mother is taking the following drugs:

Maternal drug	Effect on breastfed infant
alcohol and most anxiolytics	excessive maternal ingestion may lead to drowsiness and inhibit the infant's suckling reflex
anticoagulants	risk of neonatal haemorrhage, which is increased in the presence of vitamin K deficiency, so supplements should be prescribed with the anticoagulant; warfarin appears safe
antidepressants	the MAOIs and tricyclic antidepressants are unlikely to be harmful, but are best avoided as sedation may result; fluoxetine is secreted in significant amounts and should be avoided
anti-epileptics	barbiturates may lead to drowsiness, lethargy and weight loss in the infant with repeated doses; phenytoin is excreted in small amounts in breast milk, so monitoring of maternal plasma levels is important;

(continued)

Maternal drug	Effect on breastfed infant
anti-epileptics (*cont.*)	primidone and phenobarbital may lead to drowsiness in the infant; phenobarbital and phenytoin have had reports of methaemoglobinaemia
antimanic drugs	lithium intoxication is a potential problem, although the incidence of adverse effects is low; the risk increases with continuous ingestion so maternal and, if necessary, infant plasma concentrations should be monitored and good control achieved
antimicrobials	
• benzylpenicillin	may rarely produce allergic reactions or penicillin sensitivity
• chloramphenicol	can rarely lead to aplastic anaemia and leucopenia in the infant and is best avoided
• clindamycin	bloody diarrhoea has been reported
• nalidixic acid	haemolytic anaemia has been reported
• penicillins	the infant can develop candidiasis
• sulphonamides and co-trimoxazole	sulphonamides can lead to kernicterus*; haemolysis can occur in G6PD-deficient infants; risk of folic acid-deficiency anaemia if used long term, so haemoglobin should be checked
• tetracyclines	possibility of causing discoloration of teeth in infants
antithyroid drugs	carbimazole and propylthiouracil: breastfeeding is not contraindicated provided neonatal development is closely monitored and lowest possible doses are used; breastfeeding is contraindicated if mother is taking iodine
atropine	atropine can have antimuscarinic side-effects in the infant
fluoride	babies of mothers drinking high-fluoride water may be at risk of developing mottled teeth
hypoglycaemic agents	use should be cautious while breastfeeding, and the infant should be monitored for hypoglycaemia
hypotensive agents	infant should be monitored; large doses of diuretics may suppress lactation
laxatives	aloe, cascara and senna are all secreted in amounts sufficient to cause purgation in the infant
oestrogen contraceptives	the oral combined pill may affect lactation itself, and so should be avoided

* Kernicterus = deposition of bile pigment in the infant's brain, leading to irreversible damage.

Key points

■ Some drug metabolites require further metabolism after phase 1, for example aspirin and methyldopa.

■ Phase 2 metabolism conjugation reactions occur in the liver.

■ Some drugs, for example morphine, are further activated by phase 2 metabolism.

■ The kidneys are the most important route of drug excretion.

■ Biliary excretion of drugs is less important.

■ Factors affecting enterohepatic cycling, for example diarrhoea, can reduce the plasma concentration of some drugs, e.g. the contraceptive pill.

■ Excretion of drugs in breast milk occurs and can have an adverse effect on the breastfed infant.

Reference

1 Hale TW (2010) *Medications and Mothers' Milk* (14e). Hale Publishing. Order via Amazon.

5 The concept of a drug's half-life ($t_{1/2}$): an estimate of the rate of elimination of different drugs

Some drugs like amoxycillin are very quickly excreted, and their effective plasma concentration falls rapidly – *see* Figure 5.1. Most drugs are not eliminated so quickly – *see* Chapter 2, Figure 2.2, and with regular dosing it is possible to achieve plasma concentrations which give an optimal therapeutic response.

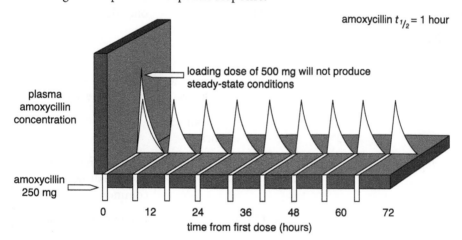

amoxycillin $t_{1/2}$ = 1 hour

plasma amoxycillin concentration

loading dose of 500 mg will not produce steady-state conditions

amoxycillin 250 mg

0   12   24   36   48   60   72
time from first dose (hours)

Figure 5.1 Peaks and troughs of plasma amoxycillin levels with multiple dosing at 8-hourly intervals.

This variability between drugs and different patients is the result of a combination of factors:

1 rate of metabolism in the liver
2 rate of excretion by the kidneys +/or intestine
3 the drug's fat solubility.

That is why defective liver or kidney function are so important to prescribers – a reduction in dosage is necessary, otherwise a build-up of drug may occur. The *BNF* often carries such a warning, particularly for elderly patients.

Table 5.1 The importance of the half-life ($t_{1/2}$) in dosage scheduling.

Drug	Short $t_{1/2}$ hours	Medium $t_{1/2}$ hours	Long $t_{1/2}$ hours	Comment
1 Antibiotics				Prescribe:
amoxycillin	~1 hr			6-hourly
oxytetracycline		~9 hrs		6-hourly
erythromycin	~1.5 hrs			6-hourly
doxycycline			~ 20 hrs	once daily
2 Angiotensin converting enzyme inhibitors (ACEIs)				Prescribe:
captopril	1–2 hrs			twice daily
enalapril		~11 hrs		once daily
lisinopril		~12 hrs		once daily
3 Sedatives/ hypnotics				
diazepam			Range 20–100 hrs Mean ~30 hrs	Prolonged sedation; may accumulate, particularly in the elderly
temazepam	5–10 hrs			Good hypnotic, but daytime drowsiness common
lorazepam		8–12 hrs		Used for treatment of epileptic fits
				Note: all sedatives and hypnotics are for short-term use only – habituation is common

~ Indicates that all $t_{1/2}$ values are approximate, dependent on individual patient factors.

During a drug's development, this variability is measured in healthy volunteers by giving a standard dose of the drug and following its plasma concentration from its peak level, at regular intervals, noting the time taken for the concentration to fall to half its peak value. That is called the drug's half-life, or $t_{1/2}$. It is a useful measure in itself, but can be extrapolated, as the plasma concentration is usually found to reduce by half again, for every $t_{1/2}$ period, so the time needed for complete elimination (or 'wash-out') can be approximately estimated.

The $t_{1/2}$ of most drugs is known and can be found in a comprehensive therapeutics textbook.[1] To illustrate its value, Table 5.1 shows the $t_{1/2}$ of some commonly used antibiotics, ACE inhibitors (for treatment of high blood pressure) and sedatives and hypnotics. Table 5.1 explains why some drugs require 6-hourly dosages while others can be taken once a day. It also shows why some chemically related drugs, the benzodiazepine group, are used as hypnotics (for sleep) – short $t_{1/2}$ – while others give 24-hour sedation for severe anxiety – long $t_{1/2}$.

This concludes the prescriber's basic guide to pharmacokinetics – 'what the body does to drugs', ADME (Absorption, Distribution, Metabolism, Excretion). Chapters 6–10 are an introduction to pharmacodynamics – 'what drugs do to the body'.

Reference

1 Hardman JG, Limbird LE and Gilman AG (2001) *The Pharmacological Basis of Therapeutics* (10e). McGraw-Hill, New York.

6 Receptor function and intercellular signalling

In Chapters 1–5 we studied pharmacokinetics: the routes of administration and the processes of absorption, distribution, metabolism and excretion of drugs, with its relevance to prescribing in primary care.

We now come to a most interesting part of modern prescribing science, concerning how drugs modify the function of body organs through their effects at the level of individual cells, namely pharmacodynamics. It is here, through advances in molecular biology, that our knowledge of drug action has expanded so greatly in the past 50 years.

Cellular society

As in human society, the infinitely complex groups of cells that form the human body succeed only so long as each individual cell participates appropriately (*see* Box 6.1).

This analogy is inadequate, however, since the cells in the healthy body live within their constraints far more precisely than people in any human society. The individual cell exists only in the context of its society, and this has probably been the case ever since the first multicellular organisms appeared some billion years ago.

Box 6.1 How healthy cells co-operate.

In good health each cell:

- performs its own specialised function adequately
- observes all the rules imposed upon it by the rest of the 'cellular society'
- accepts the communications (signals) from other parts of the same organ and distant organs
- interprets those signals correctly
- responds to those signals appropriately
- transmits its own signals to the other cells accurately.

Intercellular signalling

Cells communicate via chemical and electrical signalling. This is an immensely complex topic and only the chemical factors that are relevant to drug treatment will be described here. The relevant features of intercellular signalling are as follows:

- it is achieved by the secretion of a chemical molecule by the transmitting cell
- there are many chemical signalling molecules, including *proteins*, e.g. insulin; *amino acid derivatives*, e.g. noradrenaline, serotonin, thyroxine; *steroids*, e.g. cortisol, testosterone; *fatty acid derivatives*, e.g. the prostaglandins and leukotrienes; and *nitric oxide*
- the signalling molecule, known as the ligand, may travel far from its secreting cell, e.g. hormones (endocrine signals), may act only locally, e.g. the chemical signals controlling inflammation (paracrine signals), or may act only on a single cell across a nerve synapse, e.g. most neurotransmitters
- the 'receiving' cell recognises only the signals, or ligands, that are relevant to it: embedded in the cell membrane are a variety of proteins, some of which are receptors, with different receptors for different chemical signals
- a receptor recognises its ligand and binds it with a reversible chemical bond
- the process of chemical binding causes conformational change in the receptor protein. This change in structure activates it and leads to further signalling within the cell; this signalling in turn causes the appropriate alteration in cell function (*see* Figure 6.1)
- at any given moment throughout life, each of the multi-billion body cells will be receiving many different chemical signals. Each cell has been programmed to integrate these signals and to respond to all of its incoming information, producing an appropriate, graded response proportionate to the biological needs of the organ and organism.

The doorbell analogy

It is useful to consider receptors as similar to a doorbell (*see* Figure 6.1). There is a recognition site, the bell-button (2), which receives the external signal, pressure from the visitor's finger (1). There is a transducer site, the bell wire (3), which carries the electrical signal into the cell, the house. An effector site, the bell (4), produces an entirely different signal on the inside of the cell from that which was applied on the outside. Finally, an appropriate response (5) is evoked within the cell, just as a ringing bell evokes an appropriate response within a house.

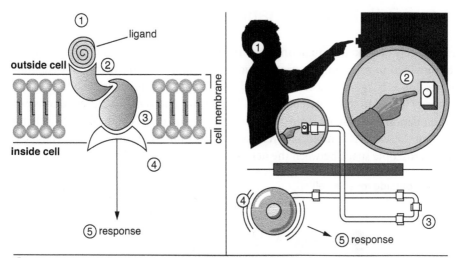

① Chemical signal (ligand) in form of drug or endogenous transmitter (person as messenger)
② Recognition site – this is the receptor protein (doorbell)
③ Transducer site – this carries the coded message into the cell (bell wire)
④ Effector site where translation of the message leads to a signal (sound of bell ringing)
⑤ Response – an appropriate action results from the signal (answering the door)

Figure 6.1 Concept of a cell receptor using the doorbell analogy.[1]

Agonists and antagonists

Many of our drugs mimic endogenous (natural) chemical signals by binding as ligands at receptors on cell membranes. Some are agonists, others are antagonists, depending on their effects at the receptor. Those drugs that initiate a response when bound to such recognition sites are called agonists, e.g. salbutamol (bronchodilator). Natural agonists include neurotransmitters, neuromodulators, growth control factors, hormones, co-enzymes and enzymes.

Those drugs that bind to such recognition sites without causing a response, but prevent access to the site by the natural agonist, are known as antagonists or receptor blockers. These are prescribed on a daily basis, for example, the beta-adrenoceptor blockers often used in heart disease.

It is important to realise that a variety of receptors are present on the surface (plasma membrane) of most cells for the purpose of receiving chemical signals.

Receptor-linked ion channels

In the receptor-linked ion channel, the recognition site, transducer site and effector are combined in one complex protein molecule. Figure 6.2 shows how skeletal muscle contraction is triggered via sodium ion channels. The sodium channel is a protein that is directly linked to the acetylcholine (ACh) receptor and remains closed to ions except on stimulation under strict regulation. This stimulation comes in the form of a chemical signal, in this case ACh molecules released from a motor neuron into the synaptic cleft (the microscopic space between the neuron and the muscle cell membrane).

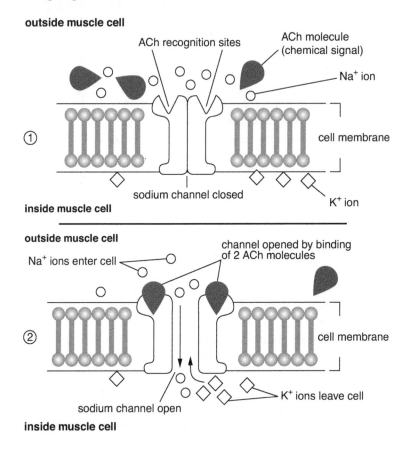

Figure 6.2 Example of a receptor-linked ion channel in skeletal muscle; the closed ion channel (1) opens in response to ACh binding (2), which leads to depolarisation of the muscle cell and initiation of contraction.[1]

Binding of the ACh molecule to the recognition site causes conformational (structural) change in the protein that forms the walls of the sodium channel (the transducer) and opens the sodium channel (the effector). Sodium ions enter the muscle cell and potassium ions leave, causing depolarisation and consequent muscle contraction (the response).

Several important muscle relaxants used in anaesthesia, e.g. pancuronium and atracurium, block the binding of ACh to the recognition site of sodium channels in skeletal muscle, in effect, a therapeutic paralysis.

Receptors linked to enzymes

The other type of effector associated with receptors is the enzyme (Figure 6.3). In Figure 6.3, note the chemical signal binding to the recognition site. This causes the transducer to activate the effector via a regulatory subunit. The effector is often the enzyme adenylate cyclase, which converts adenosine triphosphate (ATP) in the cell to cyclic adenosine monophosphate (cyclic AMP). Please note that Figures 6.2 and 6.3 are entirely schematic, to explain the different types of receptor. In reality, receptors are elongated proteins which 'weave' or 'interlace' repeatedly across the cell membrane. This anatomical/molecular reality does not lend itself readily to a succinct explanation of receptor function and has only limited relevance to the prescriber.

Cyclic AMP is an important intracellular secondary messenger, which rapidly diffuses from the membrane into the cytoplasm where it triggers a series of metabolic events leading to the final response within the cell.

Many drugs exert their effects via enzyme-linked receptors (*see* Table 6.1) and some via ion channels (*see* Table 6.2).

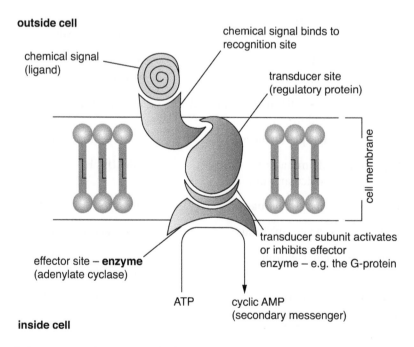

Figure 6.3 Concept of an enzyme-linked receptor (highly diagrammatic).[1]

Many receptors involve activation of a protein known as the G-protein, which is an intermediate chemical messenger. This then controls the activation or inhibition of a specific cell membrane effector. Another important secondary messenger is phospholipase C, which will not be described at present.

Table 6.1 Receptor agonists using adenylate cyclase as the effector in disease processes, and the drugs that treat them (S indicates stimulation of cyclic AMP production and I indicates inhibition; B indicates that these drugs are receptor blockers: the rest are receptor stimulators (agonists)).

	Agonist	Disease involving this agonist	Drug treatment
S	dopamine	schizophrenia – excessive dopamine	phenothiazine antipsychotics, e.g. chlorpromazine, haloperidol, fluphenazine B
		Parkinson's disease – loss of dopamine neurons	levodopa and dopamine agonists, e.g. pergolide
		hyperprolactinaemia – dopamine deficit	bromocriptine
		chemically and radiologically induced nausea, GI disorders involving spasticity, migraine, nausea	metoclopramide B
S	noradrenaline	hypertension, angina	beta-blockers, methyldopa B
S	adrenaline	asthma	salbutamol, terbutaline and occasionally adrenaline itself
S	serotonin	migraine	sumatriptan
		depression	SSRIs
S	histamine	H_1 – inflammation (allergic), motion sickness	antihistamines, cyclizine B
		H_2 – peptic ulceration	H_2-receptor antagonists B
I	prostaglandins	inflammatory disease, particularly in joints	NSAIDs B
S	glucagon	hypoglycaemia	glucagon
S	vasopressin	diabetes insipidus	vasopressin analogues
I	angiotensin-II	hypertension	angiotensin-II receptor antagonists B
I	endogenous opiates	severe pain	opioid analgesics B

Table 6.2 Drugs that exert their effect via receptor-linked ion channels.

Ion channel	Site	Drug	Effect
GABA-linked receptors	throughout brain	all barbiturates, all benzodiazepines B	from sedation to anaesthesia
5-HT$_3$ receptors (serotonin)	vomiting centre in medulla, GI tract	ondansetron, granisetron, dolasetron, etc. B	powerful anti-emetics used in chemotherapy
nicotinic ACh receptors	all skeletal muscle (at the neuromuscular junction)	pancuronium, vecuronium, etc. B	powerful muscle relaxants used in anaesthesia

GABA, gamma-amino butyric acid; B, receptor blockers.

Amplifying the signal

One important feature of receptors with enzyme system effectors is the capacity for great amplification of the original chemical signal. One extracellular signal at the recognition site can generate thousands of biochemical end-products within the cell; an example of this is the glycogen enzymatic cascade in the liver leading to the formation of glucose. Such explosive responses require tight regulation, and in all cells there are efficient mechanisms for rapidly degrading the enzyme effectors such as cyclic AMP.

It is also useful to appreciate the speed of these biochemical reactions – fractions of a second in many cases.

A similar 'cascade' causes synthesis of the prostaglandins, which are very important medically; this will be described in detail in Chapter 8. The prostaglandins are important physiological regulators but are also involved in destructive inflammatory processes.

How is the chemical signal switched off?

The majority of signal molecules are broken down (metabolised), usually by specific local enzymes, soon after binding with their receptor. This usually leads to a cessation of the intracellular response.

In the case of neurotransmitters such as noradrenaline, acetylcholine, serotonin and dopamine, the breakdown occurs in milliseconds. Excess neurotransmitter is often reabsorbed by the transmitting neuron (as, for example, with noradrenaline and serotonin reuptake). Local hormonal (paracrine) signals are broken down enzymatically within minutes, as, for example, with the prostaglandins. However, some true hormones such as cortisol and thyroxine are not metabolised for many hours.

Conclusion

This chapter has briefly covered the fundamental concepts of receptor theory. This includes where receptors are located, how the two main types of receptor work, how endogenous (natural) and exogenous chemical messengers (drugs) may activate or block receptors, and how this chemical message at the cell surface is changed to a quite different signal within the cell, sometimes with great amplification, altering cell function.

Key points

■ The human body functions only because of tight regulation of all its individual cells.

■ Regulation is achieved by continuous intercellular signalling.

■ All cells both transmit and receive signals.

■ The actual signals are chemical molecules such as noradrenaline, insulin, serotonin and prostaglandins.

■ The cell receives the chemical signal at a receptor.

■ The receptor is usually a specialised protein in the cell membrane.

■ The receptor recognition site is linked to an effector that initiates metabolic or ionic change within the cell.

■ The effector may be an enzyme or ion channel.

■ Many commonly used drugs block or stimulate these receptors.

Reference

1 Kruk Z and Whelpton R (1985) Focus on drug action. *Mims Magazine.* **April**: 1967.

Further reading (for those wishing to delve deeper into this complex and fascinating subject)

• Rang HP, Dale MM, Ritter JM, Flower RJ and Henderson G (2012) *Pharmacology* (7e). Churchill Livingstone, Oxford.
• Alberts B *et al.* (eds) (2008) *Molecular Biology of the Cell* (5e). Garland Publishing, New York and London.
• Baynes J and Dominiczak M (2009) *Medical Biochemistry* (3e). Mosby, London.

7 The central role of receptors in drug action

Continuing our exploration of receptor function and its relevance to the prescriber, it is well known that for any given intercellular signal, e.g. noradrenaline, there are a variety of different receptors, each type having a different, and sometimes opposite, function to the others. Figure 7.1 is a representation of different noradrenergic receptors and their functions in various tissue and neuronal sites.

The main purpose of this chapter is to remind readers that the response evoked by any given chemical signal depends entirely on the type of receptor to which it binds.

Noradrenaline as a physiological agonist

Figure 7.1 shows the release of noradrenaline (NA) from a neuron across a synapse. Noradrenaline may bind to $beta_1$, $beta_2$, $alpha_1$ or $alpha_2$ receptors on the postsynaptic membrane of another neuron, smooth muscle cell or cardiac muscle fibre. Each of these receptors will cause a different response in the cell when noradrenaline binds to it.

For example, in vascular smooth muscle, noradrenaline acts on $alpha_1$ receptors and causes vasoconstriction. In the smooth muscle of the bronchioles, noradrenaline acts on $beta_2$ receptors to cause relaxation.

In cardiac muscle, $beta_1$ receptors predominate and noradrenaline or adrenaline binding here will cause an increase in the rate and force of cardiac contraction.

Note the $alpha_2$ adrenergic autoreceptor in Figure 7.1. It may seem strange that a nerve ending should have built-in receptors for its own transmitter chemical. These serve as a negative feedback loop, i.e. the autoreceptors are inhibitory, and if there is a build-up of noradrenaline in the synaptic cleft, $alpha_2$ autoreceptors will inhibit further release from the neuron.

In the central nervous system (CNS), neurotransmitter action is rapidly terminated by metabolism via a specific enzyme. An example of this is monoamine oxidase (MAO), which diffuses from the surface of neuronal mitochondria and renders noradrenaline inactive. All chemical signals are metabolised to terminate their actions.

Using adrenoceptors as an example, Table 7.1 summarises their main physiological and therapeutic effects and emphasises the importance of the receptor type and its location. The predominant receptor type in any tissue will determine the effect of the chemical signal, whether it is endogenous or a drug.

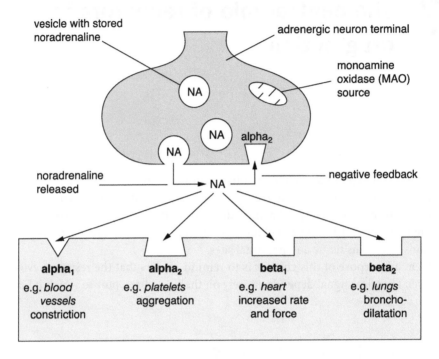

Figure 7.1 Several different receptors may exist for the same agonist; the response elicited to the agonist in a tissue or neuron depends on which receptors are present.

Receptor diversity

Although this chapter has concentrated on adrenoceptors by way of explaining the importance of the receptor rather than the chemical signal, receptors for most other physiological intercellular signals show similar, or even greater, diversity of response. The biological rationale is that a limited repertoire of chemical signals can be made to perform a very wide variety of functions.

Do not expect the nomenclature to be uniform either, as it is often based on the historical background of the original scientific discoveries and is very confusing, as Box 7.1 demonstrates.

The purpose of Box 7.1 is first to reinforce the concept that all of these subtypes may have different physiological functions and, second, to stress again that the action of any given drug depends largely on which receptor site it occupies.

Table 7.1 The effects of noradrenaline binding to different receptor types; the italics show examples of diseases whose drug treatment involves stimulating or blocking these receptors.

Tissue	Alpha$_1$	Alpha$_2$	Beta$_1$	Beta$_2$
Smooth muscle				
blood vessels	constrict (*hypertension*)	constrict (*hypertension*)	dilate	
bronchi	constrict (*asthma*)			dilate (*asthma relief*)
intestinal tract	relax			relax
non-sphincter	(hyperpolari-sation)			(no hyperpolari-sation)
sphincter	contract			
uterus	contract			relax
bladder				
detrusor				relax
sphincter	contract (*urinary obstruction*)			
seminal tract	contract			relax
iris	contract			
ciliary muscle				relax
Heart				
pacemaker			increased rate	
myocardium			increased force (*angina, hypertension, heart failure*)	
Skeletal muscle				tremor, increased contraction
Liver	glycogenolysis			glycogenolysis
Fat			lipolysis (β_3 receptor)	

(*continued*)

Tissue	Alpha$_1$	Alpha$_2$	Beta$_1$	Beta$_2$
Nerve terminals				
adrenergic		decreased neuro-transmission		increased neuro-transmission
Salivary gland	K$^+$ release		amylase secretion	
Platelets		aggregation		
Mast cells				inhibited histamine release

Box 7.1 Different receptors for common physiological signals (ligands), which are often the targets for intervention during medical drug treatment.

Example of drug treatment

Cholinergic receptors (binding acetylcholine) are subdivided into muscarinic (M) receptors and nicotinic receptors. The muscarinic receptors are divided into M$_1$ (neural), M$_2$ (cardiac) and M$_3$ (glandular).

Antimuscarinics used to treat bladder instability, e.g. oxybutynin.

Histamine receptors are subdivided into H$_1$ (bronchiolar, uterine and intestinal smooth muscle), H$_2$ (the gastric acid-secreting cells) and H$_3$ (neural tissue).

H$_2$ blockers used to reduce gastric acidity, e.g. ranitidine.

Serotonin receptors are of four types: 5-HT$_1$ to 5-HT$_4$, with several subdivisions of types 5-HT$_1$ and 5-HT$_2$.

5-HT$_3$ blockers used to treat severe nausea, e.g. granisetron.

Dopamine receptors are even more confusingly classified: there are two main types – D$_1$ and D$_2$, but D$_1$ is subdivided into D$_1$ and D$_5$, while D$_2$ is subdivided into D$_2$, D$_3$ and D$_4$.

D$_2$ blockers used to treat schizophrenia, e.g. haloperidol.

This multiplicity of receptors is the reason why some of our most important drugs have multiple, often unwanted, side-effects, as with, for example, the unselective beta-blockers (bronchospasm, cold feet), the tricyclic antidepressants (dry mouth, blurred vision, constipation, micturition problems, etc.) and the SSRIs (nausea, vomiting, dyspepsia, diarrhoea, constipation).

We have spent some time considering receptors and their functions because they are fundamental to the understanding of a large part of therapeutic drug use.

Some of the early drugs were the body's own natural (endogenous) agonists, such as adrenaline, which was used to relax the bronchioles in severe acute asthma.

However, as we have seen, the body utilises a few common chemicals but provides them with multiple actions by having different subtypes of receptor in various concentrations in different tissues. Thus, if we try to use these physiological agonists as drugs we cannot control their activity. Hence adrenaline given to relax the bronchioles in an asthma attack will also stimulate the rate and force of contraction of the heart, which can be dangerous.

However, as our understanding and discovery of the variety of receptors grew we developed synthetic drugs that were selective (or relatively selective) for different subtypes of receptor. Our understanding of receptor subtypes has revolutionised pharmacotherapy over the past 50 years.

Agonists

Although receptors are designed to be activated by endogenous ligands, they can also be activated by other molecules, particularly those with a similar structure. Armed with this knowledge, and the fact that receptors are divided into subtypes, pharmacologists set out to develop drugs that could selectively activate receptor subtypes.

A classic early example of this process was the development of isoprenaline, a drug that acted as an agonist at beta adrenergic receptors but not at alpha receptors. Following the discovery that beta-receptors were divided into $beta_1$ and $beta_2$ subtypes, and that $beta_2$ receptors relaxed the bronchioles, the $beta_2$-selective agonist salbutamol was developed. Salbutamol has been a mainstay of asthma treatment ever since. Another example of agonist drugs that act on receptors are dopamine agonists, which are used in the treatment of Parkinson's disease.

Antagonists/blockers

As well as being activated by non-endogenous drugs, receptors can also be blocked. Molecules that attach to receptors but fail to elicit a response are called antagonists. They exert their effects by blocking the action of endogenous ligands. More drugs are antagonists or blockers than agonists.

A parallel example of the therapeutic development of antagonist drugs was the initial use of the beta-blocker propranolol to slow the heart in angina. As this drug blocks both $beta_1$ and $beta_2$ receptors it can also provoke bronchoconstriction. As a result, drugs like atenolol were developed that are selective blockers of the $beta_1$ receptor, and partially spare the bronchial $beta_2$ receptors.

Selectivity is relative

Prescribers need to be clear that receptor selectivity of drugs is relative, not absolute. 'Selective' beta$_1$ antagonists have limited action on beta$_2$ receptors, so can still precipitate severe asthma. The same applies to the selective cyclo-oxygenase enzyme 2 (COX-2) inhibitor NSAIDs, which still carry some risk of gastro-intestinal (GI) and other side-effects (*see* Chapter 8). This major clinical problem applies to many drugs and is considered later (Chapter 14).

Up- and down-regulation

Receptors are not fixed in either number or the response they elicit and thus can change during long-term stimulation or blockade. In the case of agonists like salbutamol, the response to a given drug concentration diminishes, often by some form of receptor desensitisation. This is called down-regulation, which has several possible mechanisms. It is specially common in chronic pain relief with morphine, requiring ever-higher doses.

The reverse occurs on continual receptor blockade. The continued blockade of a receptor by drugs like beta-blockers causes receptor hypersensitivity to the physiological agonist, in this case adrenaline and noradrenaline. This up-regulation appears to be due to the formation of extra receptors or a shortening of the refractory phase that some receptors exhibit.

Key points

■ For a given ligand there are a variety of receptors, each of which has a different function, initiating a different cellular response.

■ Drug agonists stimulate receptor action, and antagonists inhibit it.

■ The variety of receptors can lead to unwanted adverse effects following non-specific drug agonist or antagonist treatment.

■ The newer selective agonists and antagonists are not absolute in their selectivity, and can still cause unwanted effects.

■ Long-term drug treatment can lead to up- or down-regulation of receptors, and therefore enhanced or reduced responsiveness.

---

8 Drugs that block enzymes: understanding NSAID therapy in inflammation

In Chapter 6 on intercellular signalling and receptors, we saw how a stimulatory chemical signal often releases a rapid cascade of enzymes in the receptive cell. This release of enzymes triggers a variety of biochemical changes within the cell. One of the best-understood cascades is that leading to the production of eicosanoids: prostaglandins, leukotrienes, prostacyclins and thromboxanes, which are a further stratum of important intercellular signals.

The importance of the eicosanoids can hardly be over-emphasised. Not only are they vital in the physiological regulation of many body functions, including those of the stomach, lungs, kidneys, brain, heart and genitourinary system, but they are also key players in inflammation of all types. It is in that latter role that their immense clinical importance lies.

Non-steroidal anti-inflammatory drugs (NSAIDs), which block parts of this cascade, are frequently used in general practice to control inflammation. Therefore it is important to understand how they act and why they often give problems: 30% of all serious adverse drug reactions reported annually to the UK Commission on Human Medicines are due to NSAIDs alone, including the partially selective COX-2 inhibitors.

Revising inflammation

Inflammation is normally a protective process, triggered by mechanical or microbial damage to a variety of cells – mast cells, white cells, phagocytes, lymphocytes, platelets, etc. These cells respond to damage by producing chemical signals that mediate inflammation. The chemical signals produced include some prostaglandins, histamine, various kinins, the complement system, cytokines and platelet activating factor. Box 8.1 summarises the process involved in inflammation.

All of the changes in Box 8.1 are triggered by sophisticated and controlled chemical signalling between cells, using several or all of the chemical signals mentioned above.

Let us now focus on the prostanoids. All of the components involved in the cascade are synthesised in many body cells from phospholipid in the cell membrane itself (*see*

Figure 8.1) and the 'raw material' in this process is arachidonate. Figure 8.1 is worth a moment's study, since it shows where current drugs interfere at different points in the enzymatic cascade.

Stimuli, such as an antigen/antibody reaction, cause an enzyme within the cell, phospholipase A_2, to activate. In its active form it catalyses the release of arachidonic acid from the cell membrane phospholipid into the cell.

Figure 8.1 shows why corticosteroids are such powerful anti-inflammatory agents: they block the process at step 1. In effect, they 'switch off the power at the mains'.

Once arachidonic acid has been produced, it can be used as the raw material, or substrate, for a variety of inflammatory mediators, of which only the prostaglandins and thromboxanes are shown in Figure 8.1.

The prostanoids – prostaglandins and thromboxanes

As shown in Figure 8.1, arachidonic acid is metabolised by cyclo-oxygenase enzymes (COX-1 and COX-2) to an intermediate compound (endoperoxide), which can be converted by one of two further enzymatic pathways to prostaglandins or thromboxanes. The inflammatory response is always accompanied by prostaglandin release; several prostaglandins cause potent vasodilatation of arterioles, pre-capillary sphincters and venules in many tissues.

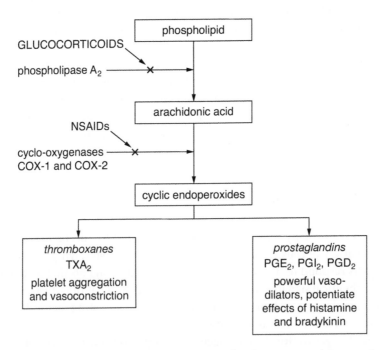

Figure 8.1 The arachidonic acid cascade is an example of an enzyme-driven pathway; the diagram shows several points where drugs block the cascade, so reducing the production of inflammatory signals.

The prostaglandins are by no means only pathological – they are part of the physiological regulation of blood flow. They also inhibit gastric acid secretion and have other physiological functions in many tissues including reproduction.[1] However, in disease they can cause trouble, nowhere more so than in the joints.

COX-1 is found in most tissues and is involved in a variety of physiological roles. COX-2, however, is only found in inflammatory cells on activation. Therefore, COX-2-specific NSAIDs are associated with fewer unwanted effects. However, there does appear to be a trade-off as there is increasing evidence of serious problems with COX-2 NSAIDs, so the decision to use these drugs should not be taken lightly. COX-2 NSAIDs should be prescribed only if the older, non-specific NSAIDs are poorly tolerated – *see BNF* warning, section 10.1.1.

The positive and negative effects of prescribing NSAIDs – non-steroidal anti-inflammatory drugs

The NSAIDs, including aspirin, all inhibit the COX-1 and COX-2 enzymes. The positive result is a dramatic reduction of joint inflammation, pain and platelet aggregation. The reduction of thromboxane A_2 (TXA_2) synthesis caused by most NSAIDs is the reason for the powerful anti-thrombotic effect of even 75 mg aspirin daily, taken to reduce the risk of coronary thrombosis.

On the negative side, most of the side-effects of the NSAIDs are due to their disruption of the prostaglandins' widespread physiological functions. In the stomach, PGE_2 inhibits acid secretion and has a protective effect on the mucosa. Therefore, the effect of NSAIDs (via COX-1) in the stomach is increased likelihood of erosion by gastric acid – the cause of NSAID-induced gastritis and peptic ulceration, often severe and fatal.

When renal circulation is impaired, prostaglandins are important in maintaining renal tubular blood flow and tubular function. That is why giving NSAIDs to elderly people with poor renal function sometimes leads to sudden deterioration of renal function and should be avoided or minimised. Box 8.2 shows the list of serious unwanted side-effects resulting from NSAID use at normal dosages – 5 are common, 3 less so.

A spin-off of research into prostaglandin physiology has been the synthesis of drugs which mimic the action of specific prostaglandins (the prostaglandin analogues). These include misoprostol, which reproduces the gastro-protective effects of (natural) prostaglandin PGE_2. Also dinoprostone, used to induce labour by reproducing the effect of PGE_2 on uterine muscle contraction, and several other specialist prostaglandin analogues used in obstetrics. See the *BNF* for further details.

Box 8.1 The process of inflammation.

Mediators of inflammation cause:

- vasodilatation, i.e. local reddening and heat; hypotension and shock can occur if widespread
- increased capillary permeability, which causes protein loss from capillaries and tissue swelling
- monocyte accumulation, which prolongs inflammation and inactivates foreign matter
- stimulation of sensory receptors, i.e. itch and pain, with protective functions
- fever, by stimulation of the hypothalamic temperature-regulation centre
- contraction of smooth muscle in the bronchioles, causing allergic asthma and, in the intestine, leading to GI pain in food allergies.

Completing the eicosanoid picture

A moment's study will show that Figure 8.1 is included in Figure 8.2, as the left-hand pathway 1. Figure 8.2 reveals how much more complex the chemical signalling of inflammation is, by including the leukotrienes, the chemotaxins and platelet activating factor (PAF). It is clear that we have a long way to go before we have the full range of drugs needed to control this complex jigsaw. Chapter 23 explores this topic.

The leukotrienes and asthma

Continuing with Figure 8.2, if arachidonate is processed by lipoxygenase (pathway 2), the end product may be a leukotriene. Like the prostaglandins, there are several leukotrienes, mostly with a physiological function. But leukotrienes are also potent mediators of inflammation – they cause more exudation of plasma from post-capillary venules than equivalent concentrations of histamine! The cysteinyl leukotrienes also cause intense bronchoconstriction, again more potent in their effects than histamine. The leukotrienes may also be the 'slow-reacting substance' of anaphylaxis (an extreme allergic reaction).

The innovation of the pharmaceutical industry has provided us with two leukotriene receptor antagonists – montelukast and zafirlukast, blocking the effects of leukotrienes in the airways. These are already useful as add-on therapy for patients with mild-to-moderate asthma which is not controlled with an inhaled corticosteroid and a short-acting beta$_2$ stimulant. We are still in the early stages of leukotriene antagonist use in medicine, and it seems relatively safe. However, the cause of the rare Churg–Strauss syndrome, a worrying adverse drug reaction comprising eosinophilia, vasculitic rash,

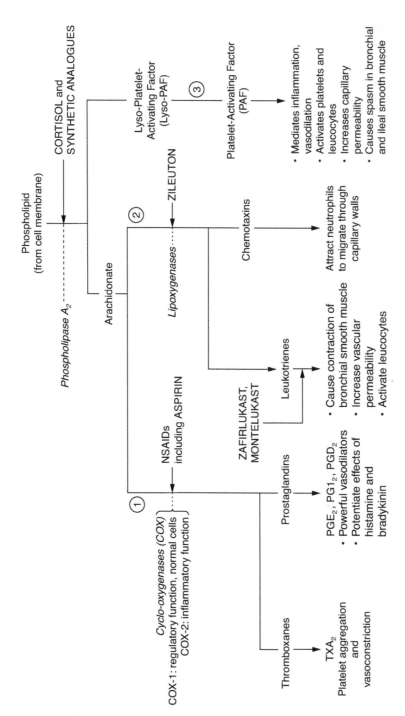

Figure 8.2 The arachidonic acid cascade: completing the picture of eicosanoid inflammatory mediators. N.B. The many physiological functions of the eicosanoids have been omitted. Enzyme-blocking drugs are shown in capitals. (Zilenton is available in the USA.)

worsening pulmonary symptoms, cardiac complications and peripheral neuropathy, may be due to the fact that our existing drugs are upsetting the balance of as yet unknown leukotriene regulation of normal function elsewhere in the body.

Box 8.2 The main serious adverse drug reactions of NSAIDs.

- Gastritis and peptic ulceration.
- Precipitation of acute renal failure.
- Loss of antihypertensive control.
- Deterioration of chronic heart failure.
- Deterioration of liver failure.
- Exacerbation of inflammatory bowel disease.
- Exacerbation of quiescent gout (in patients taking probenecid).
- Skin reactions (particularly reactivation of psoriasis).
- Loss of anticoagulation control.

Look for these side-effects whenever reviewing any patient taking NSAIDs. Few licensed drugs have such a list of serious side-effects.

An enzyme-blocking drug, zileuton, has been available for several years in the USA. This blocks the lipoxygenases, so preventing the synthesis of the leukotrienes and chemotaxins (pathway 2 of Figure 8.2).

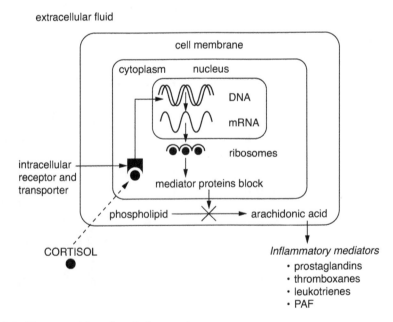

Figure 8.3 How steroids reduce inflammation.

The pharmaceutical industry is currently researching pathway 3 of Figure 8.2 for a drug which might attenuate the powerful inflammatory effects of platelet-activating factor (PAF), a major mediator of acute and chronic inflammation, including allergies.

How the corticosteroids control inflammation

When inflammation is uncontrollable by NSAIDs, as often happens in inflammatory bowel disease and rheumatoid arthritis, high potency synthetic steroids like prednisolone, betamethasone and dexamethasone are given orally. Cortisol and its many synthetic analogues act in a quite different way from all the drugs we have so far considered (*see* Figure 8.3). Steroids enter the tissue cell and are carried by a transporter molecule into the nucleus, where they activate segments of DNA to produce mRNA. This results in the production of mediator proteins at cellular ribosomes, and these proteins block the arachidonic acid cascade at its earliest point, preventing the production of all the eicosanoid inflammatory mediators (*see* Figure 8.2).

Unfortunately, prolonged oral steroid use leads to widespread steroid side-effects, including hypertension, fluid retention and depression of the immune system. That is why more specific and powerful anti-inflammatory drugs are so important, *see* Chapter 23. Taken by inhaler for moderate to severe asthma, steroids are relatively safe, as systemic absorption is low.

Other enzyme-blocking drugs

The NSAID story is the classic introduction to the drug manipulation of enzymatic cascades. The pharmaceutical industry has successfully targeted several quite different enzymatic processes, which community and hospital prescribers are now frequently manipulating to great benefit in some common and serious diseases.

1   The most obvious examples are the **angiotensin-converting enzyme (ACE) inhibitors** in the treatment of heart failure and hypertension: these block the enzymatic conversion of the inactive substrate, angiotensin I, to the potent vasoconstrictor, angiotensin II (*see* Chapter 9).
2   In the management of hyperlipidaemia, the **statins (HMG-CoA reductase inhibitors)** effectively lower LDL cholesterol with fewer side-effects than older lipid-lowering agents.
3   In treating/preventing gout, **allopurinol** blocks the enzyme xanthine oxidase, which catalyses the breakdown of purines to uric acid.
4   Recently we have seen the introduction of the **5 alpha-reductase inhibitors**, dutasteride and finasteride, an advance in the management of benign prostatic hyperplasia (BPH): they block the conversion of testosterone to the more potent dihydrotestosterone.

5 A major advance has been the advent of the **aromatase inhibitors** anastrozole, letrozole and exemestane, as adjuvant therapy for oestrogen-dependent breast cancer: they inhibit the enzyme responsible for the synthesis of oestrogen in post-menopausal women.

6 Then there is the reversible monoamine **oxidase-A inhibitor** (RIMA) moclobemide, for major depression, which reversibly inhibits the metabolism of 5-HT, noradrenaline and dopamine in cells of the central nervous system (CNS).

7 Finally, sildenafil (Viagra), tadalafil and vardenafil block the enzyme phosphodiesterase (V) leading to increased penile blood flow. It has transformed the management of male impotence.

Key points

■ Regulatory chemical signals between cells must be synthesised within the transmitter cell.

■ This synthesis usually involves one or more enzyme-dependent steps.

■ There is often an enzymatic cascade in which the same starting point (substrate) may undergo one of several enzymatic conversions, resulting in different intercellular signals.

■ The production of the prostaglandins, leukotrienes, thromboxanes and prostacyclins is a good example of this.

■ Drugs that block such enzymes halt synthesis of the products of that part of the cascade.

■ In the case of the NSAIDs, this provides powerful anti-inflammatory medications.

■ Understanding such enzymatic intracellular pathways led to the discovery of drugs that block the chemical signal themselves, for example the leukotriene receptor blockers in add-on asthma prophylaxis.

■ A further development is that of the prostaglandin analogues for therapeutic use, particularly in obstetrics, gastric acid-related disease and neonatology.

■ Modern treatment of advanced breast cancer, benign prostatic hyperplasia (BPH), severe depression, heart failure and hypertension, gout, hyperlipidaemia and erectile dysfunction are now managed by enzyme-blocking drugs.

Reference

1 Rang HP, Dale MM, Ritter JM, Flower RJ and Henderson G (2012) *Pharmacology* (7e). Churchill Livingstone, Oxford.

9   The principal targets for drug action

Not all drugs act by stimulating or blocking receptors or, as in the case of NSAIDs, enzymes. In fact, there are four main targets for drug action:

- receptors – enzyme-linked and ion channel-linked
- ion channels – voltage gated
- enzymes
- carrier molecules.

Figures 9.1–9.4 illustrate the differences between these drug targets, and carry forward the concepts of Chapters 6–8.

In each of these four cases, most drugs are effective because they bind to particular target proteins. This specificity is reciprocal: individual classes of drug bind only to certain targets, and individual targets recognise only certain classes of drug.

However, no drugs are completely specific in their actions, which is the reason for the unwanted side-effects of commonly used drugs.

For example, selective beta$_1$ blockers retain some beta$_2$ blockade activity and therefore remain a risk to asthmatic patients. Likewise, selective COX-2 NSAIDs retain some COX-1 activity and hence carry the risk of all of the NSAID adverse effects, although this risk is smaller than with the non-selective NSAIDs. COX-2 NSAIDs may also lack some of the beneficial side-effects of the non-selective NSAIDs.

Receptors as targets for drug therapy (see Figure 9.1)

Basic receptor theory has already been covered in Chapter 6. Since prescribers must frequently target receptors, it is worth looking a little further at what is currently known. Receptors can be divided into four main subtypes, each of which relates quite closely to its physiological function:

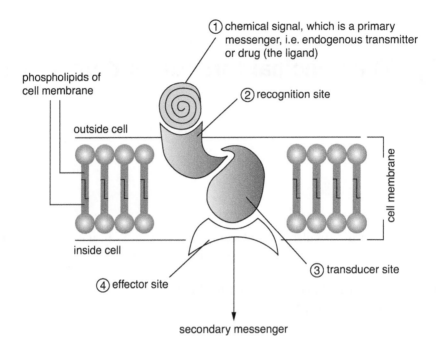

Figure 9.1a The generalised concept of a cell-membrane receptor demonstrates the process behind three of the four receptor subtypes: the drug binds to the receptor complex, triggering a series of reactions leading to the required response.

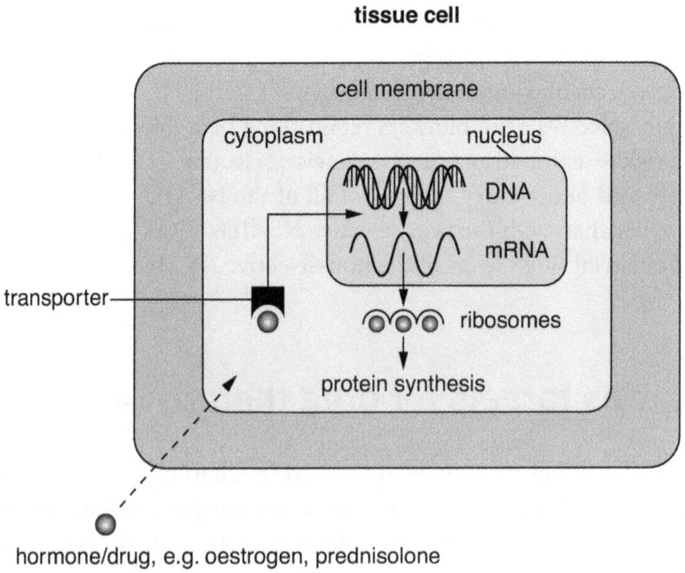

tissue cell

Figure 9.1b Steroid drugs are able to exploit nuclear receptors, the fourth receptor subtype, which act directly on DNA and affect protein synthesis.

1 The ion channel-linked cell membrane receptor. These tend to serve fast neurotransmitters in the CNS (central nervous system). They function in milliseconds, and are exemplified by the GABA-linked chloride ion channels where the benzodiazepines act.
2 The enzyme-linked cell membrane receptor, which is directly coupled to its enzyme. These channels produce their effects within minutes, and are exemplified by the insulin receptors.
3 The enzyme-linked cell membrane receptor, which is indirectly coupled via a G-protein. These produce their effects within seconds and serve many hormones and slow neurotransmitters, e.g. the adrenoceptors in the CNS.
4 Nuclear receptors linked to gene transcription, which are coupled via DNA. These produce their effect very slowly, over a period of hours or even days. Steroid hormones, oestrogens and thyroxine are examples of hormones/drugs that affect nuclear receptors, *see* Figure 9.1b. Endogenous hormones and some drugs pass through the cell membrane and attach to receptors in the cytoplasm. The receptor plus ligand complex then moves across the nuclear membrane into the nucleus. Once inside the nucleus it binds to specific parts of chromosomal DNA, resulting in messenger RNA production and protein synthesis (*see* Figure 9.1b). Steroids, oestrogen and thyroxine act via nuclear receptors, tamoxifen blocks intracellular oestrogen receptors, and slows the progression of breast malignancy.

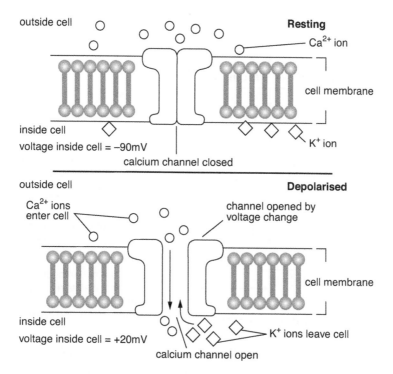

Figure 9.2 Voltage-gated ion channels open in response to a change in the voltage of the cell membrane; cardiac calcium-channel blockers, such as verapamil, block these channels.

Ion channels as targets for drug action (see Figure 9.2)

Many ion channels react to electrical rather than chemical signals. Such voltage-gated ion channels open and close in response to changes in the voltage across the cell membrane. Calcium channels in cardiac muscle are important examples (*see* Chapter 10), and the ability to block them has greatly improved the treatment of angina, hypertension and some cardiac arrhythmias.

Enzymes as targets for drug action

Many of our most important and powerful modern drugs act on enzymes in the plasma or inside cells. Their action is usually via enzyme blockade and examples include the angiotensin I-converting enzyme (ACE) inhibitors (*see* Figure 9.3). All prescribers need to be clear about the function of these important drugs.

Another commonly prescribed group of enzyme blockers are the NSAIDs, whose action and adverse drug reactions were considered in the previous chapter.

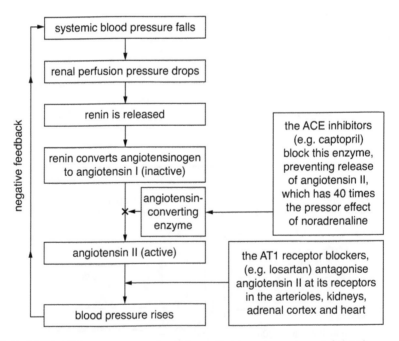

Figure 9.3 ACE inhibitors, an example of drugs that target enzymes, inhibit the production of angiotensin II, and so prevent blood pressure rising further in hypertension. The difference in action of the ACEI (enzyme blockers) and the newer angiotensin receptor (AT1) blockers is shown.

The statins are another example of enzyme-inhibiting drugs. These drugs are very valuable in cardiovascular prophylaxis and their action is now well understood. The statins competitively inhibit an important enzyme involved in cholesterol synthesis in the liver (HMG-CoA). This action effectively lowers LDL-cholesterol with fewer side-effects than the older lipid-lowering agents. The statins have been proved to reduce the risk of heart attack and death in patients with angina, and following a heart attack or stroke.

Allopurinol is useful in the treatment of chronic gout because it blocks the enzyme xanthine oxidase, which catalyses the final breakdown of purines to form uric acid.

A further example of enzyme-blocking drugs is the monoamine oxidase inhibitor (MAOI) group, which are still used occasionally in cases of depression that have not responded to other agents. The serious side-effects of the MAOIs are well known, and are due to blockade of the enzyme outside the CNS.

Other enzyme blockers include the aromatase inhibitors (e.g. anastrozole), used as part of the treatment of breast cancer, and finasteride, used to treat benign prostatic hyperplasia.

Carrier molecules as targets for drug action

As mentioned earlier in the book, ions and less lipid-soluble molecules are transported in and out of cells by carrier proteins. These carrier molecules play an important role in the excretion of drugs by the renal tubule, which was described in Chapter 4. Among the most commonly prescribed drugs in primary care are several that block carriers.

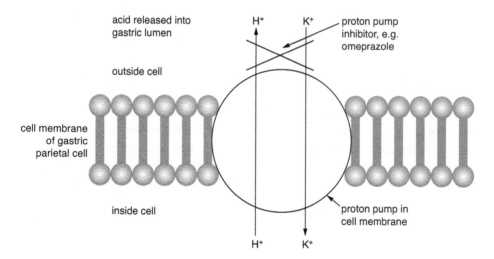

Figure 9.4 Omeprazole, which is a proton pump inhibitor, inhibits carrier molecules transporting ions in and out of cells in the gastric mucosa, and hence prevents gastric acid (H^+Cl^-) synthesis.

1 The **proton pump inhibitors,** e.g. omeprazole, block the H^+/K^+ exchanger in the gastric mucosa (*see* Figure 9.4).
2 The **loop diuretics** block the $Na^+/K^+/2Cl^-$ co-transporter in the (renal) loop of Henle, greatly reducing water reabsorption.
3 **Digoxin** blocks the Na^+/K^+ pump in cardiac muscle, slowing heart rate and increasing its force of contraction.
4 The tricyclic antidepressants block the carrier mechanism responsible for the reuptake of the neurotransmitter noradrenaline from the synaptic cleft of brain neurons.

Conclusion

It is hoped that this chapter will have given readers a clear concept of the varied mechanisms by which different prescribed drugs achieve their therapeutic benefit. Table 9.1 shows the four most significant cellular targets of some important drugs prescribed in primary care.

It is worth noting that with every new drug discovery has come a better understanding of molecular biology, which in turn has led to more precise focusing of the search for safer and more effective drugs.

Table 9.1 Examples of drugs acting at the four targets for drug action.

Target	Effect (clinical use)	Effect (clinical use)
Receptor	**Agonist**	**Antagonist**
beta receptor	dobutamine (shock)	beta-blockers, e.g. propranolol (hypertension and angina)
histamine H_2 receptor	histamine	ranitidine, etc. (suppression of gastric acid)
opiate receptor	morphine (pain relief)	naloxone (opiate overdose)
5-HT_3 receptor	serotonin	ondansetron, etc. (severe nausea)
dopamine D_2 receptor	dopamine (Parkinson's disease)	chlorpromazine, etc. (schizophrenia)
oestrogen receptor	ethinylestradiol } contraception	tamoxifen (breast cancer)
progesterone receptor	norethisterone } contraception	danazol (endometriosis and benign breast disease) via pituitary gland

(*continued*)

Target	Effect (clinical use)	Effect (clinical use)
Ion channel	**Stimulator**	**Blocker**
Na$^+$ channel in renal tubule	aldosterone	amiloride, triamterene (fluid overload)
voltage-gated Ca^{2+} channel in heart and arterioles	no drug	dihydropyridines (e.g. nifedipine, etc.) (hypertension and angina)
ATP-sensitive K$^+$ channels in pancreatic B cell		sulfonylureas (e.g. gliclazide, etc.) (diabetes)
GABA-gated Cl$^-$ channels in CNS	benzodiazepines (anxiety and insomnia)	flumazenil (benzodiazepine overdose)
Enzyme	**Enhancer**	**Inhibitor**
COX-1 and COX-2		NSAIDs, e.g. ibuprofen (inflammatory arthritis)
ACE		ACE inhibitors, e.g. captopril (hypertension and heart failure)
HMG-CoA reductase		statins, e.g. simvastatin (hypercholesterolaemia)
dihydrofolate reductase		trimethoprim (urinary infections)
DNA synthetases		azathioprine (immunosuppressant)
5 alpha-reductase		finasteride (benign prostatic hyperplasia)
aromatase		anastrozole, etc. (breast cancer)
Carrier	**Accelerator**	**Inhibitor**
noradrenaline reuptake	amphetamines	tricyclic antidepressants (depression)
serotonin reuptake		SSRIs (depression)
'proton pump' (H$^+$/K$^+$-ATPase)		proton pump inhibitors, e.g. omeprazole (suppression of gastric acid)
cardiac 'Na$^+$/K$^+$ pump'		cardiac glycosides, e.g. digoxin (cardiac arrhythmias)
renal tubular ion carriers		all diuretics (fluid overload)

Key points

- There are four known targets for drug action.
- A drug may act at either a receptor, an ion channel, an enzyme or a carrier mechanism.
- Drugs acting on enzymes or carrier mechanisms have mostly been discovered in the last 30 years.
- They include drugs to block enzymes involved in inflammation, excess cholesterol, advanced breast cancer, benign prostatic hyperplasia and erectile dysfunction.
- Drugs acting on carrier mechanisms include the diuretics and drugs to treat depression, peptic ulceration and heart disease.
- A table summarises the four drug targets, with examples of each type of drug and its common clinical uses.

10 Calcium ion for the prescriber

As we have already seen, some of the most important chemicals involved in cell signalling are simple ions such as potassium, sodium, calcium and chloride. Calcium ion is one of the most important of these, modulating cellular metabolism, so its concentration in the cell cytoplasm is very strictly regulated. Box 10.1 gives a list of the main functions of calcium ion.

Box 10.1 The main functions of calcium ion.

- Regulates muscle contraction – smooth, skeletal and cardiac muscle.
- Regulates the release of many neurotransmitters and hormones.
- Regulates/controls permeability of cell membranes to other ions.
- Regulates the activities of many intracellular enzymes.
- Has 'secondary messenger' functions (secondary messengers are intracellular mediators, e.g. between a receptor and an enzyme; *see* Chapter 6).
- Depolarisation of many excitable tissue cells, including most nerve terminals.
- Programmed cell death (apoptosis) – an essential feature of tissue repair, immunity and development.

Because of the importance in primary care of calcium-channel blockers such as nifedipine, the rest of this chapter will concentrate on item 1 in Box 10.1 – regulation of muscle contraction. Muscles will not contract without calcium ion, whether they be smooth, skeletal or cardiac. Calcium ion does two things in the muscle cell:

1 it activates the sequence which produces the energy for muscle contraction – ATP/ADP, without which there can be no contraction
2 it activates the cross-bridging between actin and myosin in muscle cells, which is the process by which chemical energy is transformed into mechanical energy.

The reason why we can use calcium-channel blockers to control cardiac dysfunction without affecting skeletal muscle function is that the source of calcium ion for muscle contraction varies between the three muscle types:

1 *Heart muscle* – calcium enters heart muscle from the extracellular fluid in a controlled way via voltage-sensitive L, N and T calcium channels (*see* Figure 10.1). This is the so-called 'slow calcium current' (*see* Figure 10.2). The L-type channels predominate in the general heart muscle, the myocardium, while the T-type channels occur mainly in the sino-atrial node (the pacemaker), and the conducting tissues of the heart.
2 *Vascular smooth muscle* – calcium ion enters from the extracellular fluid via L and T calcium channels and further calcium is recruited from intracellular stores.
3 *Skeletal muscle* – calcium is released from intracellular stores (the sarcoplasmic reticulum). Cell membrane calcium ion channels are not involved.

Clearly, calcium-channel blockers will affect heart muscle and vascular smooth muscle, but not skeletal muscle.

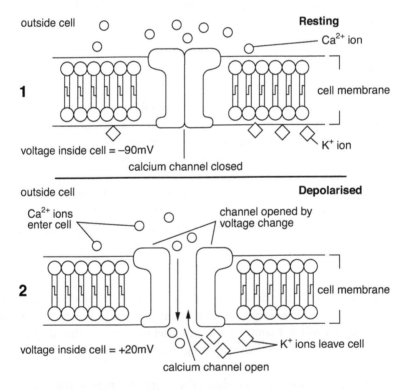

Figure 10.1 The voltage-gated ion channel as a drug target. Calcium enters heart muscle from the extracellular fluid via the voltage-sensitive L, N, and T calcium channels, which open in response to depolarisation.

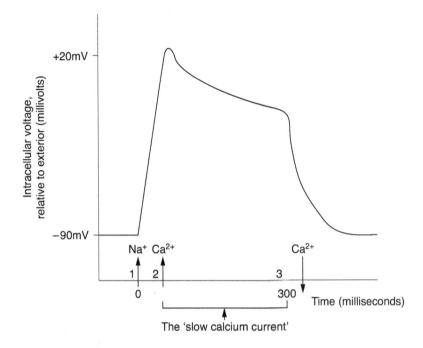

Figure 10.2 The electrical and ionic events of cardiac contraction. (1) Initial rapid depolarisation, caused by opening of voltage-gated Na^+ channels. (2) Slower, prolonged opening of voltage-gated Ca^{2+} channels, resulting in contraction. (3) Repolarisation by extrusion of Ca^{2+} by Ca^{2+} pump mechanisms. (1)–(3) includes the QRST of the classical ECG. *The clinical ECG is not helpful in understanding the action of cardiac drugs.*

How do calcium-channel blockers work?

When the cell membrane of a cardiac or smooth muscle cell undergoes voltage change (depolarisation), the voltage-gated calcium ion channels in the membrane open. This allows calcium ion to enter the cell from the extracellular fluid, initiating the sequence of contraction. Calcium-channel blockers, such as nifedipine, bind selectively to these calcium channels only in their closed phase, maintaining closure and preventing calcium ion from entering the cell. This reduces the force of contraction, leading to a reduction of cardiac work and increased peripheral arteriolar vasodilation, with a reduction in hypertension (via blockade of calcium ion entry to the smooth muscle cells of the arterioles), i.e. a valuable dual action.

Table 10.1 shows the main pharmacological differences between the three main groups of calcium-channel blocker, with their relative therapeutic benefits.

Table 10.1 Choosing the right calcium-channel blocker depends on its predominant site of action.

Drug	Concentration of its recognition sites	Resulting useful therapeutic effects
Nifedipine	Peripheral vascular smooth muscle +++	• Strong hypotensive effect
	Coronary smooth muscle ++	• Anti-anginal effect
	Cardiac muscle +	• Little reduction in contractility
	Cardiac pacemaker/conductors +	• Weak conduction effect
		Overall: relatively safe in general practice
Verapamil	Peripheral vascular smooth muscle ++	• Good hypotensive effect
	Coronary smooth muscle ++	• Anti-anginal effect
	Cardiac muscle ++	• Reduces contractility*
	Cardiac pacemaker/conductors +++	• Strong conduction effect**
		Overall: use with caution in general practice
Diltiazem	Peripheral vasculature +	• Good hypotensive effect
	Coronary vasculature ++	• Good in vasospastic angina
	Cardiac muscle ++	• Reduces contractility*
	Pacemaker/conductors +++	• Strong conduction effect**
		Overall: use with caution in general practice

* liable to precipitate heart failure

** liable to cause conduction disorders

Why are the nifedipine group (the dihydropyridines) so safe?

As every clinician knows, there are major differences in the uses and safety margins between the three main types of calcium blocker – the nifedipine group, verapamil and diltiazem. The best current explanation for this is that only the L-type channel is sensitive to the nifedipines (the dihydropyridines). Now, L channels predominate in the smooth muscle of the peripheral arterioles, maintaining the appropriate level of arteriolar constriction to regulate blood pressure in normal health. In hypertension, the nifedipine group of calcium-channel blockers cause excellent, sustained peripheral vasodilation by L-calcium-channel blockade in the arteriolar smooth muscle. Cardiac contractility is also reduced somewhat, but the sympathetic baroreceptor reflex is sufficient to maintain cardiac output. Into the bargain, all members of the nifedipine group powerfully dilate the coronary vessels. Hence, we have a very useful therapeutic package, whose main side-effects are a consequence of the primary drug action – flushing and peripheral oedema. Look up the *BNF*, section 2.6.2, to learn the unpleasant side-effects of these important cardiac drugs.

Table 10.2 Therapeutic differences of the dihydropyridines.

Drug	*Comment*
Nifedipine (the original DHP)	Does all that is required, safely, but must be given in sustained-release (SR) form – its short half-life leads to reflex tachycardia between doses. H, A
Nicardipine	Equally good, with fewer side-effects. Should also be given in SR form. Decreases the frequency of angina and improves exercise tolerance in exercise-induced angina. H, A
Amlodipine*	As effective as nifedipine, but its long half-life (>36 hours) reduces the risk of reflex tachycardia. H, A
Felodipine*	An even better peripheral vasodilator than nifedipine, and has negligible depressant effect on heart muscle. H, A
Isradipine	Produces good peripheral vasodilation. Selectively inhibits the cardiac pacemaker (SA node), eliminating reflex tachycardia – the so-called negative chronotropic effect. Has no effect on the general myocardium. Can be used with beta-blockers in appropriate circumstances. H only
Nimodipine	Its high lipid solubility allows it to enter the CNS, hence it is used to relax destructive cerebral vasospasm following subarachnoid haemorrhage.

H = for hypertension; A = for prevention of angina

* Often prescribed in preference to the older drugs nifedipine and nicardipine, as they do not reduce myocardial contractility.

Verapamil and diltiazem – use with care!

Why do verapamil and diltiazem depress cardiac contractility and conduction so much more powerfully than the nifedipine group of calcium-channel blockers (*see* Table 10.1)? Currently, the best theory is that after cardiac contraction, the calcium ion which entered the muscle fibre at the start of contraction must be pumped out again, into both the extracellular fluid (by the Na^+/Ca^{2+} pump) and the cardiac intracellular calcium store (by the ATP-dependent calcium pump). Both verapamil and diltiazem delay this recovery process (repolarisation), but members of the nifedipine group do not – *see* Figure 10.2.

Of major clinical importance, it has recently been found that the effects of both vera-pamil and diltiazem are enhanced when the heart rate rises (in exercise or fear), leading to a profound negative inotropic effect (reduction of strength of contraction) and a high risk of precipitating heart failure. This effect is not seen with the nifedipine group of calcium-channel blockers so in primary care, the benefits and safety of this group are obvious. That being so, it is well worth knowing the relative advantages of the different dihydropyridines available to the prescriber: they are by no means identical in action. Table 10.2 summarises the differences and suggests relative indications. The decision to prescribe verapamil or diltiazem should be shared with a consultant cardiologist.

What of the T-calcium ion channels?

As described above, T-calcium channels are present mainly in the cardiac conducting tissue. The pharmaceutical industry is currently searching for a safe, selective calcium T-channel blocker which would have the advantage of reducing the activity of the cardiac pacemaker and protecting the diseased heart from rate increases due to adrenergic stimuli resulting from emotional and other stresses. This should make T-channel blockers particularly useful in hypertensive patients with angina.

Left ventricular hypertrophy and calcium ion

Finally, left ventricular hypertrophy (muscle thickening) is associated with excess retention of calcium ion within cardiac muscle. Verapamil alone, of the older L-calcium-channel blockers, is effective in normalising cardiac function in such cases, though ACE inhibitors appear to share this important effect. In addition, verapamil may reduce hypercalcinosis in hypertensive arterial walls. Further, secretion of aldosterone by the adrenal medulla is dependent on T-calcium channels. These are all good reasons for treating moderate-to-severe hypertension with calcium-channel blockers, for left ventricular hypertrophy is present in 20% of all hypertensive patients, greatly worsens their prognosis, and is often missed on ECG. Hypertensive patients with other risk factors such as hyperlipidaemia, obesity and a history of smoking should be referred for echocardiography. Regression of left ventricular hypertrophy can be achieved in its early stages by prompt management of the hypertension which causes it.

Key points

■ The main functions of calcium ion are listed.

■ The chapter then focuses on the role of calcium ion in muscle contraction.

■ The voltage-gated calcium ion channel is described.

■ Calcium ion is a key feature of cardiac contraction.

■ Different calcium-channel blockers have stronger or weaker effects on the different parts of the cardiovascular system.

■ Understanding these differences helps the prescriber to select the optimal drug in each patient.

■ The enlargement (hypertrophy) of the wall of the left ventricle is associated with excess retention of calcium ion.

DRUGS AND THE CENTRAL NERVOUS SYSTEM

11 Introduction to drugs in the central nervous system

The human central nervous system (CNS) comprises the entire brain and spinal cord. It is the most complex thing in the observable universe, and while we can describe its structure in detail, our knowledge of its functions is very limited. If the human brain were a 1000-piece jigsaw, then current knowledge amounts to about 50 pieces! For the rest, we have weakly supported theories upon which to base our drug treatments, e.g. of depression or schizophrenia. One reason for this is that we cannot experiment directly on the human brain; another is its extreme complexity. Extrapolation from animal studies is often the best we have.

Knowledge of drug action in the CNS has often been gained as follows, over the past 65 years.

1 It is noticed that a drug given for another illness (e.g. an antihistamine or an antituberculous drug) relieves the symptoms of psychiatric disease (e.g. schizophrenia or depression).
2 Laboratory animal studies are done to determine which receptors the drug acts upon; these often involve 'sacrificing' the animal to perform cellular and biochemical assays on its CNS.
3 It is then postulated that these must be the receptors whose function is disturbed in the human patient.
4 A painstaking search begins for chemical variants of the original drug, seeking greater potency (effectiveness per milligram), greater safety and fewer adverse effects.

That is how most of our best antidepressants and antipsychotics and our current theories began life in the 1950s. Our knowledge will certainly increase over the next 50 years, probably quite slowly. All of which may seem unsatisfactory, but it does not stop us treating CNS illness effectively. For all the lack of cogent theory, drug treatment of psychiatric illness has improved greatly since 1950.

So our lack of knowledge is the first starting-point in these chapters. The second is that you need to understand Chapters 6–9 of this book before proceeding. Chapters 6–9 will be referred to as appropriate. Although much CNS illness (neurology and psychiatry) should be supervised by a specialist, team management is now the effective approach to long-term care. All team members likely to be prescribing or giving CNS drugs should understand what is known about them, and the theories regarding what is not known.

As an introduction, let us look at three things:

1   the nature of nerve-cell signalling and where drugs act (targets)
2   the main types of neurotransmission
3   the principal CNS neurotransmitters.

The main CNS drug targets

The hundred billion nerve cells (neurons) in the CNS can serve their functions (sensory perception, control of movement and posture (motor activity), memory, thought and emotions) only because they are in continuous highly integrated and co-ordinated communication with each other. Each neuron may have as many as 1000 active communication terminals called synapses, so the potential for sophisticated information transfer is, in computer terms, at the billion gigabyte level.

Synapses are important in the present discussion, because most of our useful CNS drugs – analgesics, anxiolytics, antidepressants and antipsychotics – act at or around the inter-neuronal synapse. As Figure 11.1 shows, the two neurons are not in direct contact and signal transmission is by means of the neurotransmitter, a chemical synthesised in the pre-synaptic (transmitting) neuron, which is released into the gap between the neurons (the synaptic cleft) and binds chemically to a receptor site on the post-synaptic (receptive) neuron, where this chemical binding either stimulates or inhibits the receptive neuron.

The pre-synaptic neuron and its supporting cells have carrier mechanisms (*see* Chapter 9) which reabsorb the transmitter (neurotransmitter reuptake). This 'switches off' the signal.

It is probable that many effective antidepressant drugs work by inhibiting reuptake of neurotransmitters like serotonin (SSRIs) and noradrenaline (tricyclics) (Figure 11.1 – compare Figure 7.1, p. 44).

Our antipsychotic drugs appear to work by inhibiting the release of another neurotransmitter, dopamine, in certain brain nuclei. Conversely, the 'recreational' CNS stimulant drugs like the amphetamines and cocaine cause massive release of dopamine in some brain areas. Our best treatment for Parkinsonism is the supply of dopamine to the motor-regulation area of the brain, where it is severely deficient in such patients.

The powerful opiate pain relievers (analgesics), like morphine and diamorphine, bind strongly to the opioid receptors which appear to control ('gate') the transmission of painful stimuli to the conscious level (*see* Chapter 15).

Some drugs used to control nausea and vomiting (anti-emetics) act as blockers (antagonists) of dopamine or serotonin at the zone in the CNS which triggers vomiting (the chemoreceptor trigger zone, or CTZ) (*see* Chapter 16).

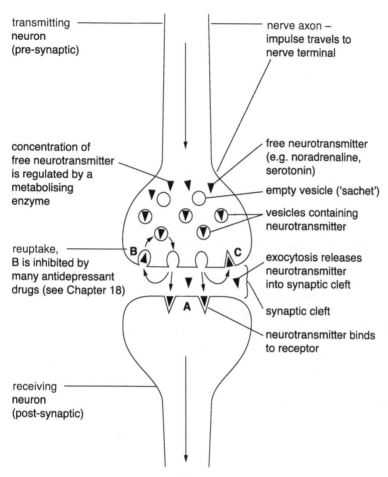

transmitting neuron (pre-synaptic)

nerve axon – impulse travels to nerve terminal

concentration of free neurotransmitter is regulated by a metabolising enzyme

free neurotransmitter (e.g. noradrenaline, serotonin)

empty vesicle ('sachet')

vesicles containing neurotransmitter

reuptake, B is inhibited by many antidepressant drugs (see Chapter 18)

exocytosis releases neurotransmitter into synaptic cleft

synaptic cleft

neurotransmitter binds to receptor

receiving neuron (post-synaptic)

Figure 11.1 Simple schema of a nerve synapse. A, neurotransmitter binds to receptors on the receiving neuron, stimulating or inhibiting a nerve impulse; B, excess neurotransmitter is 'captured' by the empty vesicle (reuptake) and 'recycled'; C, neurotransmitter may bind to an autoreceptor (i.e. a receptor on the transmitting neuron) (*see* Chapter 7).

Our best sedatives, the benzodiazepines, stimulate inhibitory neurons throughout the brain.

All of these, the antidepressants, the antipsychotics, the anti-anxiety drugs (anxiolytics), the anti-Parkinsonism drugs, the analgesics and the anti-emetics, will be described in succeeding chapters. Before that, it is important to have a concept of the time/distance factor in neurotransmission, i.e. the duration of action of a neurotransmitter and the range of its activity (its 'domain' or territory).

The main types of neurotransmission – fast, slow and distant

Many important neurotransmitters act on a 1:1 inter-neuronal basis, as Figure 11.2 shows. Their neuron-to-neuron signalling is fast, specific and individual. It occurs within milliseconds on a receptor less than half a micron away and ceases as quickly, with reuptake of the neurotransmitter. Examples are the neurons signalling voluntary movement, or visual input from the retina. Other equally important neurotransmitters with different functions are relatively slow, acting over hundreds of milliseconds at receptors on several neighbouring neurons. They probably modulate the levels of neuronal activity, e.g. the fine tuning of motor (movement) signals – a process known as neuromodulation (*see* Figure 11.2).

Third, there are distant neurotransmitters with quite prolonged diffusion times and durations of action, acting on dozens of neurons relatively far from the originating neuron. These may represent a half-way house in neuronal signalling, between true neurotransmitters and local hormones. Some of these are thought to have a role in memory.

The reason for mentioning these variants is that they are probably all involved in complex syndromes like depression, where some 'totality of brain integration' expresses 'personality'. (A cogent theory awaits its Nobel prize!) At the level of current drug treatment of depression, it is almost certain that networks of interdependent neurons are intimately associated, and it is highly unlikely that a drug could affect one such network without causing changes in the others. The extensive side-effects of all psychotropic drugs (drugs affecting mood and behaviour) are evidence in support of this statement.

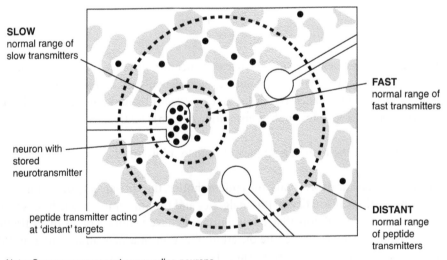

Note: Grey areas represent surrounding neurons

Figure 11.2 Slow, fast and 'distant' neurotransmitters in the CNS.

Table 11.1 Neurotransmitters, drugs affecting them, known effects of these drugs and diseases treated by them.

Neurotransmitter (alternative name)	Receptor type	Drug group(s) affecting	Example drug(s)	Known effects of drug	Disease(s) treated
Noradrenaline (Norepinephrine)	Noradrenergic and serotonergic (non-selective)	Tricyclic antidepressants (TCAs)	amitriptyline	Effective antidepressant: augments effects of noradrenaline and serotonin by blocking reuptake	Depression and agitated depression (has a sedative effect)
Serotonin (5-hydroxytryptamine, 5-HT)	Serotonergic (5-HT) selective	Selective serotonin reuptake inhibitors (SSRIs)	fluoxetine (Prozac)	Effective antidepressant; augments effects of serotonin	Depression (less sedating than TCAs)
	Serotonergic ($5\text{-}HT_3$) in CNS	'Setron' anti-emetics – $5\text{-}HT_3$ antagonists	ondansetron	Powerful anti-emetic. Blocks $5\text{-}HT_3$ receptors in chemoreceptor trigger zone (CTZ) in CNS	Extreme nausea and vomiting, e.g. in cancer chemotherapy
	Serotonergic ($5\text{-}HT_4$) in intestine	Gastro-intestinal $5\text{-}HT_4$ receptor agonists	metoclopramide	Stimulates peristalsis-controlled gastro-intestinal propulsion	Non-ulcer dyspepsia and gastro-oesophageal reflux (GORD)
	Serotonergic ($5\text{-}HT_{1A}$)	CNS $5\text{-}HT_{1A}$ partial agonists	buspirone	Delayed-action anxiolytic	Specialist management of anxiety
	Serotonergic ($5\text{-}HT_{1D}$)	CNS $5\text{-}HT_{1D}$ agonists – the 'triptans'	sumatriptan	Vasoconstriction of arteries throughout the body – may precipitate angina	Acute migraine and 'cluster' headaches
	Serotonergic ($5\text{-}HT_1$)	Ergotamine group (alkaloids) $5\text{-}HT_1$ antagonists	ergotamine	Vasoconstriction of arteries throughout the body. Also raises BP by stimulating alpha-adrenoceptors – a risky drug	Specialist management of migraine and 'cluster' headache prophylaxis (prevention)
Dopamine	Dopaminergic D_2	All antipsychotic drugs	flupentixol olanzapine	Antagonise excess dopamine release from amygdala and other CNS centres	Schizophrenia – remove many symptoms and sedate without impairing consciousness
	Dopamine, noradrenaline and serotonin receptors	All amphetamines and related drugs are highly unselective agonists at all these receptors	dexamphetamine MDMA cocaine methylphenidate (Ritalin)	Cause intense release of dopamine, noradrenaline and serotonin in CNS and inhibit their reuptake / Unknown mode of action	Strongly addictive 'recreational' drugs / Attention deficit/hyperactivity disorder in children – specialist use
			fenfluramine	As for dexamphetamine	Appetite suppressant – not in BNF

(continued)

Neurotransmitter (alternative name)	Receptor type	Drug group(s) affecting	Example drug(s)	Known effects of drug	Disease(s) treated
Dopamine (cont.)	Dopaminergic D_2 receptors in CTZ	Dopamine D_2 receptor antagonists	metoclopramide and domperidone	Block dopamine D_2 receptors in chemoreceptor trigger zone (CTZ) – see Chapter 16	Powerful anti-emetics and gastro-intestinal peristaltic stimulants – see serotonergic action above
	Dopaminergic neurons in substantia nigra of CNS	Levodopa, given always with a dopa-decarboxylase inhibitor (see Chapter 14)	co-careldopa co-beneldopa	Replenish dopamine deficit in movement regulation centre of CNS	The mainstay of treatment of Parkinsonism
Opioid peptides	μ (mu) opioid receptors	All morphine-like (opioid) mu-receptor agonists in the CNS; also at spinal cord level (suppressing upward transmission of pain stimuli)	morphine diamorphine methadone fentanyl, etc . . .	Cause hyperpolarisation of pain centre neurons, thus inhibiting release of their pain-sensation impulses to higher centres – see Chapter 15. Also act in spinal cord, suppressing upward transmission of pain stimuli to brain	The most powerful analgesics known. Also have a beneficial euphoric effect, e.g. in terminal disease. Often cause severe nausea and severe respiratory and cardiac depression. All are very addictive
	μ (mu) opioid receptors	Opioid antagonist	naloxone	Displaces all opiates from the mu receptors throughout the body and so reverses all opiate effects	Opiate overdosage, given intravenously. Highly effective and life-saving, but has a much shorter half-life than the opiates and must be repeated if signs of opioid overdose recur
Glutamate	NMDA ion channel	NMDA channel blockers	ketamine	Blocks fast excitatory neuronal transmission in CNS	Short-acting intravenous anaesthetic, useful in children. May cause post-anaesthetic psychotic symptoms – hallucinations
GABA (gamma-aminobutyric acid)	$GABA_A$	All benzodiazepines Benzodiazepine antagonist	diazepam temazepam midazolam flumazenil	Sedative Hypnotic Deep sedation Benzodiazepine antagonist	Anxiety Insomnia Day procedure anaesthetic Benzodiazepine overdose

Lastly, although signalling between neurons is chemical, the nerve impulse stimulated by the chemical signal is electro-chemical – it involves a wave of electrical depolarisation travelling along the neuron's surface. Any basic physiology text will explain this process in detail.

A few important CNS drugs act on enzymes or cell transport mechanisms (*see* Chapter 9).

The principal CNS neurotransmitters known to be affected by neurological, psychiatric and 'recreational' drugs

Bearing in mind our ignorance of the physiology and biochemistry of most illnesses associated with the CNS, it is necessary only that the prescriber should be aware of the neurotransmitters' names, with the briefest mention of the known effects of the commonly used drugs (*see* Table 11.1). Their general action and the disease(s) they are used to treat, reading across from the left column to the far right column, are individually described in greater detail in subsequent chapters. The reader should spend 15 minutes studying Table 11.1, because all of these ranks and columns will be expanded in the remaining chapters of this CNS section. This table supplies as much background on drug action (pharmacodynamics) as most primary care prescribers probably need, and it includes most of the CNS drug groups in current use. Since we are intervening in patients' brain function whenever we prescribe such drugs, it is essential that we have as clear a concept of their action as limited modern knowledge can provide.

Note how only six neurotransmitters can serve so many functions. This biological economy is achieved by developing several different receptors for the same neurotransmitter (*see* Chapter 7), each receptor having a very different function to its 'relatives'. Our knowledge of receptors has often followed from the discovery of new drugs and investigation of their novel effects.

Key points

- Problems in understanding brain disease and drug action are introduced.
- Brain neuronal function is described.
- The main neurotransmitters, their receptors, the drugs which affect them and the diseases these drugs treat are summarised in a table, as an introduction to Chapters 12–21.

12 CNS drugs whose action is (a) understood, (b) unknown/ speculative

Drugs whose action is understood

Our knowledge of drug action in the CNS began through the astute observation of clinicians that drugs used for entirely different purposes had certain beneficial effects on mental illness. That stimulated the intensive research and development of the past 65 years, with the discovery and study of drugs known to alleviate anxiety, depression, schizophrenia, etc., including what is now known of their action (pharmacodynamics). Chapters 13–16 will look at drugs whose action we feel confident about. Chapters 17–20 will describe drugs which are effective, but whose action is largely speculation – theory, with some evidence for and against. The final chapter (Chapter 21) deals with what we know about Alzheimer's disease. Do not begin this section without careful study of Chapter 11 and revision of Chapters 6–9.

We have an adequate understanding of the following therapeutic areas:

- drugs used to treat anxiety, insomnia and status epilepticus (Chapter 13)
- drugs used to treat Parkinsonism (Chapter 14)
- drugs used to treat severe pain and migraine (Chapter 15)
- drugs used to treat nausea and vomiting (Chapter 16).

Drugs whose action is unknown/speculative

Although we have effective drug treatments for schizophrenia, depression and epilepsy and we know what receptors these target in animal preparations, we can only guess what they may do in the human brain. This book is about 'how drugs work', and if that is not known, all that is needed is a summary of what *is* known and what current theories are. That is not without value, because new antidepressant and antipsychotic drugs are usually marketed by a trumpeting of their *supposed* pharmacodynamics. Do not be misled! And always challenge such animal-study assertions. Perhaps in a decade or two we may have some 'hard evidence' of their action in man. For the present, we must be very grateful to have antipsychotic, antidepressant and anti-epileptic drugs, which daily transform the lives of many millions around the globe. Study Chapter 11 carefully before beginning this section.

Because of the increasing prevalence of mental illness caused by so-called 'recreational' drugs – drugs of addiction and habituation – there is a final chapter in this section supplying what is known; again, rather vague and poorly supported theory.

We have an incomplete understanding of the following areas:

- antipsychotic drugs (Chapter 17)
- antidepressant drugs (Chapter 18)
- anti-epileptic drugs (Chapter 19)
- 'recreational' drugs (Chapter 20)
- Alzheimer's disease (Chapter 21).

Key points

■ The action of many effective neurological and psychiatric drugs is not known.

■ Chapters 13–16 deal with those diseases where drug action is understood.

■ Chapters 17–21 deal with those diseases where drug action is speculative.

13 The actions of CNS drugs used to treat anxiety, insomnia and life-threatening status epilepticus

'Although these drugs are sometimes prescribed for stress-related symptoms, unhappiness or minor physical disease, their use in many situations is inappropriate.'
BNF, 2014, 66: 4.1.2

Management of anxiety revolves around an adequate diagnosis – is the patient's anxiety sufficient to require drug treatment, is it generalised, or panic or a phobia or post-traumatic? If it is, then drug treatment should be accompanied by skilled psychotherapy, the elements of which can be readily learnt. In the early drug treatment of anxiety, the benzodiazepines are effective and safe, and we know how they work.

To understand benzodiazepine action, we need to consider the CNS transmitter molecule gamma-aminobutyric acid (GABA), which inhibits neuronal activity throughout the CNS. A GABA molecule binds to $GABA_A$ receptors which are linked to chloride ion (Cl^-) channels in the cell membrane of CNS neurons (*see* Figure 13.1). This binding causes the Cl^- channel to open, which allows Cl^- ion to enter the neuron from the extracellular fluid; that hyperpolarises the neuron, making it insensitive (refractory) to further stimulation, as long as the Cl^- channel remains open. So GABA always inhibits the neuron whose receptor it occupies. The drugs most often prescribed for severe anxiety and insomnia, the benzodiazepines, all bind to a separate site on the GABA-linked Cl^- channel (*see* Figure 13.2). Their effect is indirect insofar as they enhance GABA inhibition of neurotransmission, i.e. they potentiate GABA. They are relatively non-toxic because they do not act at all Cl^- channels – only those controlled by GABA.

Medium- or long-term use of benzodiazepines is to be avoided, because they cause some habituation and dependency in vulnerable people, though not true addiction. They should be seen as a short-term aid to the management of anxiety. That may allow the less severely affected patient to recover, as often happens in primary care. If not, the patient requires third-level care which may involve other CNS drugs like tricyclic antidepressants (TCAs).

Benzodiazepines are excellent hypnotics, but their sleep-promoting properties are short-lived: habituation occurs within a week, after which ever higher doses are needed to get any sleep. They should always be used for a few nights only and be accompanied by instructions as to behaviour modification of the sleep pattern. Patients may be given a small supply to use intermittently. One or two doses may be helpful in short-term insomnia due to shift work, noise and jet-lag, for a few nights only.

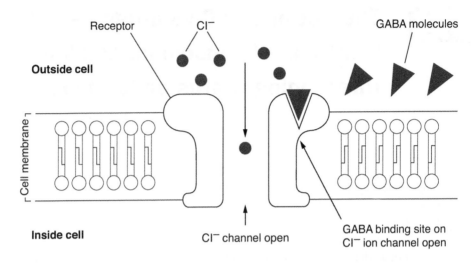

Figure 13.1 Gamma-amino butyric acid-A (GABA$_A$) receptor in the central nervous system. Cl$^-$ = chloride ion.

The intravenous benzodiazepine lorazepam is the treatment of choice in acute, severe epilepsy (status epilepticus). Diazepam rectal solution is a good substitute if the convulsions prevent IV access. Benzodiazepines have no place in anti-epileptic prophylaxis – *see* Chapter 19.

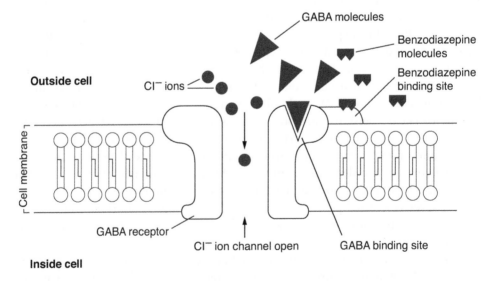

Figure 13.2 The interaction of benzodiazepines and central nervous system GABA$_A$ receptors. GABA = gamma aminobutyric acid; Cl$^-$ = chloride ion.

Types of benzodiazepine

The original benzodiazepine, diazepam, marketed as 'Valium', was a true breakthrough. As the drug industry enthusiastically researched this discovery, many molecular variants were spawned, and it was discovered that small chemical changes in the original molecule resulted in widely differing clinical applications (*see* Tables 13.1 and 13.2). Yet they all share the action at the GABA$_A$ receptors. Most of the differences are due to the variant drug's duration of action (the half-life or $t_{1/2}$) (*see* Chapter 5), but some are more specific, e.g. their action being due to an active metabolite of the drug produced in the patient's liver.

Table 13.1 Anxiolytics/sedatives.

Name	Half-life (hrs)	Approved uses according to the British National Formulary (BNF)
Benzodiazepine anxiolytics		
diazepam	20–40	*Oral:* Short-term relief of severe anxiety. Must never be used alone in depression or agitated depression (suicide risk). Causes drowsiness, giddiness and staggering (ataxia), and confusion, especially in the elderly. Other side-effects – *see BNF*
		Intravenous: Status epilepticus*, panic attacks, acute alcohol withdrawal. Always use the emulsion (Diazemuls)
		Rectal: Where the oral or intravenous route is unavailable (absorption is rapid)
		Benzodiazepines are of no value in preventing epilepsy
lorazepam oxazepam	8–12	*Oral:* Short-term relief of severe anxiety. Similar side-effects to diazepam. Useful in patients with impaired liver function
		Intravenous: IV lorazepam is now the preferred treatment of status epilepticus
Non-benzodiazepine anxiolytics		
buspirone		Short-term relief of anxiety but takes up to 2 weeks to act. Best used with specialist consultation. Inhibits serotonin (5-HT$_{1A}$) receptors and some CNS noradrenaline receptors
beta-blockers		Reduce tremor and palpitations but have no effect on worry, tension or fear. Action – *see* Chapter 7. Tense snooker players have found them helpful because of the physical effect of reducing tremor!

* Status epilepticus = epileptic fits lasting more than 5 minutes, jeopardising respiration.

Table 13.2 Hypnotics/sleep-inducing drugs.

Name	Half-life (hrs)	Approved uses according to the British National Formulary (BNF)
Benzodiazepine hypnotics		
loprazolam	8–12	Short-term use (1 week) as hypnotics and anxiolytics
lormetazepam		Cause a few hangover effects
temazepam		Withdrawal effects common if use is prolonged
nitrazepam flurazepam	16–30	Short-term use (1 week). All cause drowsiness and giddiness next day, with amnesia. Cause confusion and staggering (ataxia) in the elderly. Dependence develops rapidly
diazepam	20–40	Occasionally useful as a single dose at night, where the insomnia is associated with daytime anxiety. Sedation continues well into the next day, due to long-acting metabolite nordiazepam
chlordiazepoxide	20–40	First line management of alcohol withdrawal
Non-benzodiazepine hypnotics		
zaleplon	1	These have few advantages over the benzodiazepines. They act on the same GABA$_A$ receptors. For short-term use only
zolpidem	2	They have many more side-effects than the benzodiazepines
zopiclone	4	Occasionally useful in elderly patients but not routinely. Relatively free from hangover effects
clomethiazole	5	Second-line management of alcohol withdrawal

Note that chronic insomnia is rarely helped by hypnotics and is often due to dependence caused by injudicious hypnotic prescribing, or to other psychiatric illnesses like depression, anxiety or drug or alcohol abuse (*BNF*, 2004).

Treatment of the underlying condition usually cures the insomnia. The short notes in the *BNF* on anxiety and insomnia should be regularly re-read by everyone using these drugs. There are other hypnotics and anxiolytics, but only those approved for NHS prescribing are included in Tables 13.1 and 13.2.

Afterthought: It is easy to start a patient on a benzodiazepine. It is often very hard to get him or her to stop.

Benzodiazepine overdose

Benzodiazepines are very safe, even in very high doses. Where there is concern about severe overdosage, third-level care (A&E) specialists may give intravenous flumazenil. That drug is a competitive antagonist – it reverses the effect of benzodiazepines at the $GABA_A$ receptor (*see* Figure 13.2). Flumazenil is also used by anaesthetists to reverse the anaesthetic effect of the short-term benzodiazepine midazolam used in minor surgery.

Always remember, when co-prescribing any anxiolytic or hypnotic, that it will potentiate the effects of other CNS depressants that the patient is taking, including alcohol.

Key points

■ The need for adequate diagnosis of anxiety is stressed.

■ The $GABA_A$ chloride ion channel is described.

■ The action of the benzodiazepines in treating anxiety and insomnia is described, with reference to the $GABA_A$ chloride channel of neurons.

■ Two tables summarise the different benzodiazepines and their approved uses.

■ The drug treatment of benzodiazepine overdose is outlined.

14 Drugs used to treat Parkinsonism

In this distressing and very common condition, we know what is wrong and we know what our treatments do to rectify it. To begin with, here is a brief description of the underlying physiology and what disrupts it in Parkinsonism.

Co-ordinated voluntary movement is the result of the close-coupled integration of many parts of the brain starting with the cerebral cortex, where the decision to move is made and where the movement initiation centre (the motor cortex) signals that intention to the 'lower' centres responsible for its execution. These include the thalamus, the globus pallidus, the corpus striatum and the substantia nigra with intense input from the cerebellum (*see* Figure 14.1). These anatomical names are historical and have no functional meanings, but in Figure 14.1 you will recognise three neurotransmitters from Chapters 11 and 7.

This system acts in highly controlled sequence to plan and programme all voluntary movements so that they are smooth, fluid and of exactly the right extent (amplitude). It also ensures that movements start and stop promptly and that each movement is co-ordinated with balancing movements of many muscle groups throughout the body.

In Parkinsonism, all of these functions are progressively impaired; there is coarse tremor at rest and excessive muscle tone (rigidity of all muscle groups), movements are slow to start and slower to stop and co-ordination with other muscle groups is poor. Hence the 'classical' symptoms needed for a certain diagnosis of Parkinsonism:

- tremor at rest, often seen first in the fingers and thumbs
- muscle rigidity
- slower movement
- progressive postural instability.

As the condition worsens, all of these become more marked until, in the terminal stages, the patient is almost immobile and can barely speak – a most distressing condition. Late in the disease, dementia is common, and before that happens, depression is often present, since the intellect is unimpaired and the patient is well aware of his or her plight.

The planning and programming system in Figure 14.1 consists of three feedback loops, A, B and C. Note the GABA neurons, the dopamine neurons and the acetylcholine (cholinergic) neurons of loop C, for that is where the pathology is in Parkinsonism. Progressive death of dopamine neurons in the substantia nigra (black diamond) leads to a progressive deficit of the neurotransmitter dopamine (1). This results in a loss of inhibition of the excitatory cholinergic neurons of the corpus striatum (2). These nerve fibres discharge excessively in regular bursts, causing the coarse tremor of Parkinsonism. The GABA neurons of the corpus striatum are stimulated by these cholinergic signals to send inhibitory signals to the GABA neurons of the globus pallidus (3). That prevents them from sending inhibitory signals to the thalamus (4), which is thus deprived of the information needed to serve the stopping, starting, speed, amplitude and evenness of movement.

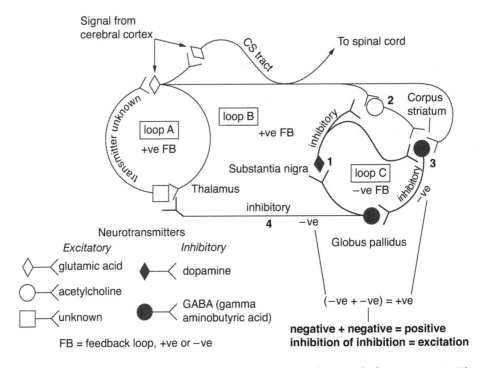

Figure 14.1 CNS nuclei and nerve pathways concerned with control of motor activity. This scheme is based on available anatomical, physiological and pharmacological data; though a gross oversimplification, it is useful in understanding the nature of Parkinson's disease.

Since Parkinsonism is caused by lack of dopamine in loop C, replacement of dopamine should relieve the symptoms, and that is what is done for tens of thousands of patients, every day.

Dopamine is supplied as the 'pro-drug' levodopa, which is metabolised to dopamine in the brain, where it relieves the symptoms of Parkinsonism effectively, in the early stages. There are two major problems with levodopa. First, less than 1% of an oral dose reaches the brain. The remainder is metabolised to dopamine in many body tissues, giving many intolerable side-effects. The drug industry has overcome this problem by combining levodopa with either of two other drugs which inhibit the peripheral breakdown of dopamine and ensure that a sufficient amount reaches the CNS. These adjuvant drugs are carbidopa and benserazide and there is little to choose between the two combination preparations, co-careldopa and co-beneldopa. Both reduce the tremor and rigidity, in most patients.

The second and so far insuperable problem is that levodopa does not stop the progression of the disease, and the effectiveness of the drug declines in line with that. Worse than that, levodopa gives rise to serious CNS side-effects, often within two years. These are involuntary movements of the face and limbs (dyskinesia) and the aptly named 'on–off' effect, which is a vivid description of normal functioning (the 'on' period) and sudden onset of weakness and restricted mobility (the 'off' period). There is sometimes a gradual deterioration, as cerebral concentrations of dopamine decline (the 'end-of-dose effect').

Much research has gone into improved treatments which have all been beneficial, but disappointing in comparison to levodopa. They include selegiline, and rasagiline, which reduce the metabolism of dopamine in the brain by inhibiting one of its metabolic enzymes, monoamine oxidase-B (MAO-B). Selegiline may be used as 'add-on' therapy to levodopa. The other enzyme which metabolises peripheral levodopa is catecholamine-O-methyltransferase (COMT). Entacapone inhibits COMT, allowing more levodopa to reach the substantia nigra in the brain to reduce the 'end-of-dose' deterioration. For specialist use only.

Other drugs are those which stimulate the remaining substantia nigra dopamine receptors (agonists) and are sometimes used in early Parkinsonism, to delay the start of levodopa therapy. These include ropinirole, rotigotine and pramipexole. Unfortunately, they also stimulate dopamine receptors generally and have many unpleasant side-effects, some seriously anti-social. A further group of drugs, the anticholinergics, block the excessive excitatory action of the cholinergic neurons in the corpus striatum (2 in Figure 14.1). These include trihexyphenidyl, orphenadrine and procyclidine, but they are for specialist use only, to counter the adverse Parkinsonian effects of antipsychotic drugs used long-term to treat schizophrenia.

Treatment of Parkinsonism should not be started until symptoms disrupt the quality of life and should always be planned by a specialist.

Finally, it is important to remember that because all of the anti-Parkinsonism drugs are unselective, they act wherever their target appears in the body. Consequently they all have many unpleasant side-effects. However, none of these are as intolerable as the symptoms of the disease itself. Acceptance of unpleasant drug side-effects by patients often depends on this type of balance in many conditions, e.g. cancer chemotherapy.

In advanced Parkinson's disease, all the major features of the disease can be relieved, or greatly improved, by chronic bilateral electrical stimulation of the thalamus or globus pallidus (*see* Figure 14.1). That is done by implanting fine electrodes by stereotactic surgery, carried out in several UK specialist centres. Transplantation of stem cells into the corpus striatum holds promise but remains semi-experimental.

Late-stage Parkinsonism

In its later stages, much more widespread and unpleasant symptoms indicate that the neurological damage includes much more than the motor control centres described above. These include psychiatric symptoms – depression, anxiety, dementia, apathy and sleep disturbance. Other distressing symptoms are loss of bladder control, constipation and, in men, erectile dysfunction.

Finally, it must be stressed that the management of PD should be consultant-led from the start. First, there are 16 conditions to be excluded before a firm diagnosis of PD is established. Second, its successful drug treatment demands specialist familiarity with the choice of drug combinations, all of which have serious risks and side-effects: see *BNF*'s nine pages of prescribing guidance – section 4.9.1.

Key points

- The pathology of Parkinsonism and its diagnosis are described.
- A figure outlines the neuronal deficit of Parkinsonism.
- The use of levodopa combinations to replace the dopamine deficit is described, together with their limitations.
- The newer anti-Parkinsonian drugs are described.
- The problems of late-stage PD are described.

15 Pain and analgesics

Pain is a complex phenomenon, particularly in humans. The following is a description of current understanding of pain, and of evidence-based theory as to its 'auto-regulation' by the CNS.

1 Pain results when tissue damage of any type stimulates the sensory endings through-out the body of small, non-myelinated nerve fibres (C-fibres) with low conduction velocities. These are often known as the C-polymodal nociceptors (PMN). These fibres have a high response threshold and are normally activated only by intense stimuli. C-fibre activity causes a dull burning pain, while other fibres (A-fibres) cause sharp, well-localised pain.

2 The initial cause of pain, e.g. nettle sting, burn, abrasion – results in the local release of cell-signalling chemicals such as 5-HT and bradykinin, lactic acid, ATP, K^+ ion and several of the prostaglandins. It is believed that these chemical agents act on the nerve terminals, activating them directly or enhancing their sensitivity to other forms of stimulation. Note that injury causes release of inflammatory prostaglandins from the injured tissue area. Prostaglandins increase the responsiveness of the PMN (C-fibres) to these chemicals. NSAIDs block this effect, hence their action as mild analgesics (*see* later and Chapter 8).

3 The C-fibres themselves produce substances which actually promote inflammation by their effects on blood vessels and cells of the immune system. This is known as neu-rogenic inflammation, which amplifies and sustains the local inflammatory reaction and activates nociceptive (pain) nerve endings in the region. These 'neuropeptides' are substance P and calcitonin gene-related peptide (CGRP).

4 Acute and chronic pain are very different; acute pain occurring in an otherwise pain-free individual is not self-generating. Chronic pain, on the other hand, is accom-panied by hyperalgesia (an increased perception of pain from the same stimulus), allodynia (pain evoked by a non-noxious stimulus) and spontaneous spasms of pain without any precipitating stimulus. Everyone has experienced both hyperalgesia and allodynia with every first-degree burn or bee sting.

5 The gate control theory of pain sensation (*see* Figure 15.1) states that peripheral pain fibres (1) run with other sensory nerves into the posterior (dorsal) horn of the spinal

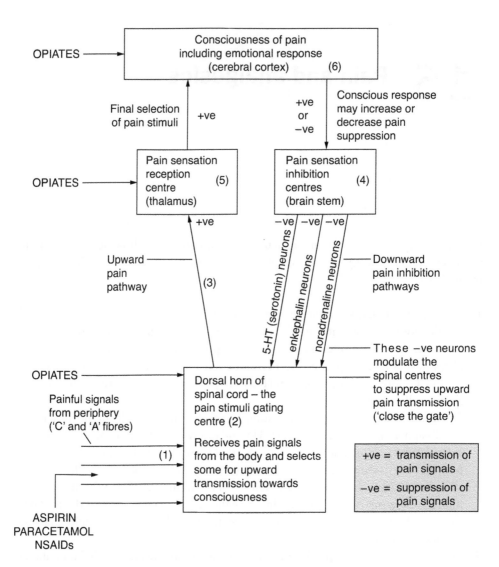

Figure 15.1 Simplified scheme of pain pathways and their autoregulation. Analgesic drugs are shown in capital letters.

cord and synapse with spinal cord neurons which are programmed to transmit the more intense pain signals to the brain centres, or to withhold them. This has been called 'gating' (2). It is probable that hyperalgesia is caused by 'opening of the gate', allowing signals which were previously suppressed to reach the brain. Transmission of painful stimuli from the spinal cord to the thalamus is inhibited (gated) by these dorsal horn neurons in the spinal cord so that only persistent C-fibre activity will be transmitted to the brain in the spinothalamic (upward) nerve pathway. Hence, successive bursts of activity in the nociceptive neurons become increasingly effective in activating the transmission neurons (3).

6 The brain itself can 'shut the gate' and so reduce the intensity of pain signals it receives. It does this through powerful descending control systems (Figure 15.1) (4). A series of specialised brain nuclei interrelate to exert an inhibitory influence on transmission from the spinal cord, via at least two pathways, the one releasing enkephalins, the other releasing serotonin (5-HT) (4). A third, separate system releasing noradrenaline has a similar activity. The actions of morphine and other opioids are also indicated in Figure 15.1.

7 The subjective nature of pain is evident from the fact that, besides conventional analgesics such as the opioids and NSAIDs (including aspirin) and the local anaesthetics, the antidepressants appear to have a pure analgesic action in patients who are not suffering from depression but who are suffering from pain. It is possible that monoamine transmission is involved.

8 Other specific analgesics treat the cause of the pain, e.g. ergotamine and sumatriptan, 5-HT_{1D} agonists in the treatment of migraine.

9 The sensation of pain is probably located in the thalamus (5) but is modulated by the sensory cerebral cortex (6) which adds affective, discriminatory and motivational dimensions to the thalamic sensation. The brain also produces morphine-like chemicals (opioid peptides) which strongly inhibit the transfer of pain signals to the conscious level, in a manner resembling morphine.

10 Pain due to damage to the pain-receiving pathway (e.g. chronic pressure by a slipped disc in the spine or tumour infiltration) (neuropathic pain) is a special form of pain which is not easily controlled even by opiates. This presents a major problem for doctors and nurses involved in palliative care, 'back clinics', shingles and diabetic neuropathy.

11 Other endogenous neurotransmitters are involved in pain sensation, but their role is still being researched.

How pain-relieving drugs (analgesics) are thought to work

Morphine and its near relation diamorphine (heroin) are the strongest analgesics known, still unsurpassed in making bearable the unbearable. Pharmaceutical research has synthesised codeine (a moderate analgesic) and pethidine, fentanyl (useful in its transdermal patch formulation), methadone (useful in managing heroin addicts), pentazocine and buprenorphine (Nalbufen, used by paramedics). But none of these are as effective as morphine and diamorphine, though they each provide a 'step' on the 'analgesic staircase'.

The opiates work centrally in the mid-brain nuclei and the cerebral cortex (causing feelings of well-being and tranquillity, termed euphoria). They stimulate release of 5-HT, noradrenaline and enkephalins to close the spinal dorsal horn 'gate', and they act directly to inhibit the spinal dorsal horn and further inhibit the peripheral terminals of the C pain fibres. They inhibit pain signals at every level – *see* Figure 15.1.

Three opioid receptors have been identified, named by the Greek letters mu (μ), delta (δ) and kappa (κ). They are all targets for the endogenous (natural) opioids (the enkephalins), but morphine and other opiate analgesics bind very selectively to the μ receptor.

An excellent short account of the clinical uses of the opiate analgesics is to be found in the *BNF*, Chapter 4 and 'guidance on palliative care', giving pros and cons, differing delivery formulations, doses and side-effects. N.B. Tables of equivalent dosages of the main opioid analgesics in *BNF* 'Guidance on Prescribing'.

Side-effects of opiate analgesics

All prescribers need to be acutely aware of the serious side-effects of the opiates, some of them life-threatening. They occur in all patients, but the risk is greatest in opiate-naïve people (whose receptors are unaccustomed to opiates). They are fully described in the *BNF*, but the most serious are respiratory and cardiac depression, severe constipation and prolonged drowsiness (coma in patients with liver failure). Nausea and vomiting are common and can be severe but not life-threatening, so morphine is often injected in combination with an anti-emetic (*see* Chapter 16). Tolerance and dependence develop rapidly, due to downregulation of the cell membrane receptors (Chapter 7).

Morphine is a most important aid to good palliative pain relief. It is very well tolerated and the dose may be increased many times over several weeks, as symptom-control demands. N.B. The use of drugs in palliative/terminal care is a highly specialised branch of therapeutics, in which many community nurses and GPs become expert and share care.

Opiate overdosage

This is most often seen in diamorphine (heroin) addicts and is now very common. Naloxone, given intravenously, displaces opiates from the μ binding sites, rapidly reversing all the toxic effects but also removing the analgesic effect. The half-life of naloxone is only 30–40 minutes and it must be repeated if the opiate toxicity is not to return (morphine has a $t_{1/2}$ of 4–5 hours and will re-occupy the μ receptors as soon as the naloxone molecules have left) – *see also* Chapter 25.

Analgesics for mild and moderate pain

Aspirin and paracetamol, the oldest synthetic pain relievers, are still the commonest drugs for self-medication. Surprisingly their pharmacodynamics (modes of action) are not known! They are effective in moderate headache, muscle pains and arthritic pain, but little use for visceral pain. They have a weak NSAID effect (see below). Paracetamol is very toxic in overdose, while aspirin has many side-effects, including tinnitus (ringing ears), vertigo, nausea, vomiting, gastrointestinal bleeding, and acute asthma in asthmatic patients.

The non-analgesic benefits of aspirin taken in low dose and long-term have been studied and proven, particularly its antiplatelet action, reducing the risk of coronary thrombosis and of its recurrence, and its reduction of the risk of colorectal cancers. The dosage of aspirin for such prevention is much lower than for pain-relief (*see* the *BNF*) – 75 mg daily.

The NSAIDs. From the discovery of ibuprofen in the early 1970s in Nottingham, NSAIDs have revolutionised the management of moderate pain due to tissue inflammation, particularly inflammatory arthritis. They have been described in Chapter 8. The 26 different NSAIDs vary in both analgesic and anti-inflammatory potency and in the severity of many side-effects which they all share, including gastro-intestinal perforation and haemorrhage, acute renal failure and asthma (*see* Box 8.2). *See also* Chapter 22.

How drugs work in migraine

The management of acute migraine (a blinding one-sided headache which usually incapacitates the patient for its duration) has been revolutionised by the discovery of the drug family the triptans, of which sumatriptan was the first. They may be taken as tablets, injections (subcutaneous), or nasal spray. They are agonists (stimulants) at the 5-HT_{1D} receptors in the brain. Unfortunately, the pathophysiology of migraine is still unknown – another example of our ignorance of much CNS function (described in Chapter 11). It is known that cerebral blood flow is altered in certain migraine attacks. Triptans have no place in the prophylaxis (prevention) of migraine. Drugs are used for prevention in severe cases only (two or more acute migraines per month). They include a beta-blocker (*see* Chapter 7), a tricyclic antidepressant (*see* Chapter 18), or a newer drug, pizotifen, which blocks histamine (an inflammatory amine released during inflammation) and is a serotonin receptor antagonist. See the *BNF*, 'prophylaxis of migraine', for more details. As in acute migraine drug treatment, the mode of action of these effective prophylactics in preventing the neurophysiological disorder causing migranous headache is unknown.

Key points

- The origin of pain at the tissue level is described.
- The pain pathways to and from the conscious level are outlined in a figure and described in detail.
- The 'gate control' theory of pain is outlined.
- The sites of action of morphine and the other opiate drugs in relieving pain (analgesia) are shown.
- Drugs for mild and moderate pain are outlined, together with their many adverse effects.
- A paragraph describes drugs used to treat migraine.

16 How anti-emetic drugs work

The management of nausea and vomiting is particularly important in cancer chemo-therapy and palliative care. It is sometimes necessary post-operatively, in pregnancy and to prevent motion sickness. The treatment of severe nausea has been greatly improved in the past two decades and this chapter aims to describe the actions of anti-emetic drugs in the CNS and gut. To do that, it is necessary to describe the two relevant control centres in the brain stem, the vomiting centre and the chemoreceptor trigger zone (CTZ). These are outside voluntary control and both of them react to a variety of nauseant stimuli (*see* Figure 16.1).

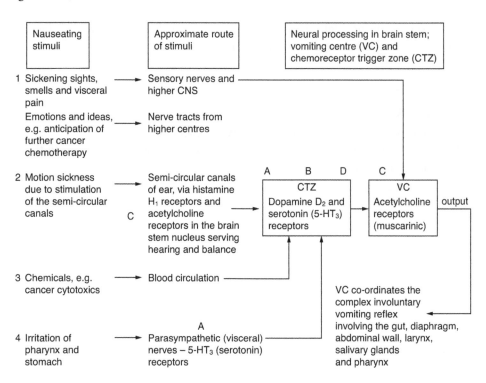

Figure 16.1 Pathways controlling nausea and vomiting in the CNS.

Please study Figure 16.1 carefully for a few minutes, as understanding it makes explanation of the pharmacology of anti-emetic drugs quite straightforward. We already understand the function of receptors (Chapters 6 and 7) and the commoner CNS receptors (Chapter 11). The capital letters A, B, C . . . on Figure 16.1 indicate where the anti-emetic drugs have their effect. They all stimulate or block one or more specific receptor(s).

- A – The most powerful anti-emetics, granisetron, ondansetron and palonosetron, are selective $5\text{-}HT_3$ antagonists. They block $5\text{-}HT_3$ receptors particularly in the CTZ, but also in the intestine.
- B – Metoclopramide and domperidone are both dopamine D_2 receptor antagonists acting in the CTZ. Metoclopramide has the advantage of also being 'prokinetic', i.e. it is a specific stimulant (agonist) of the $5\text{-}HT_4$ receptors in the gastro-intestinal tract which promote peristalsis (emptying of stomach contents in a downward direction!).
- C – The much older histamine H_1 receptor antagonists block H_1 receptors peripherally, as well as in the CNS. They also have a selective anticholinergic effect, which adds to their value as mild anti-emetics. The commonest drug is cyclizine. This group of drugs is often useful in treating vertigo due to inner ear (cochlear) disease; their action here is unknown.
- D – The antipsychotic drugs, the phenothiazines (e.g. prochlorperazine) are useful anti-emetics, as antagonists of the dopamine D_2 receptors in the CTZ.

In very severe vomiting, high-dose synthetic steroids like dexamethasone may be used, under specialist supervision. Their action is unknown.

Key points
- The physiology of nausea and vomiting is described.
- The actions of all the main anti-emetic drugs are shown in relation to the known physiology.

17　Antipsychotic drugs

The psychoses (psychotic illnesses) all involve serious disturbances of brain function at its higher levels. These may include disruption of thinking, behaviour, social relationships, speech, sensation and, often, mood. Schizophrenia is the most serious of the psychoses and it will be referred to solely in this chapter. However, the other psychoses respond to drugs which improve schizophrenia. Any clinician suspecting a psychosis should refer the patient immediately to a psychiatrist, for the diagnosis and management of psychotic illness is now a highly specialised field.

The dopamine theory of schizophrenia rests mainly on indirect (and conflicting) evidence that schizophrenic patients have more than double the normal concentration of dopamine in several brain nuclei, such as the amygdala, which, in animals, appear to be the centres responsible for rage and aggression.

The second and somewhat complementary theory of schizophrenia is the glutamate theory. This is even more tenuous, resting on the observations that drugs which block glutamate receptors in humans (e.g. the intravenous anaesthetic drug, ketamine) cause psychotic symptoms, and also, that there are reduced glutamate concentrations in schizophrenic brains (at post-mortem).

The dopamine–glutamate theory is another 'gate' theory. It is suggested that the two types of receptor are in a delicate balance, preventing 'unnecessary' sensory overload of the cerebral cortex, thus stopping it from reaching consciousness. Underactivity of the excitatory glutamate neurons or overactivity of the inhibitory dopamine D_2 neurons (it is suggested) disrupts the gating mechanism and allows inappropriate sensory input to higher centres.

These theories are probably far too simplistic, for we do not know the neurological basis of personality, which is at the centre of schizophrenia. I say that because all the antipsychotics bind to several other receptors as well as dopamine D_2 receptors, e.g. 5-HT_2, histamine H_1 and alpha-adrenergic neurons – quite a repertoire! Table 11.1 indicates that all the antipsychotic drugs strongly antagonise (block) dopamine D_2 neurons. They also antagonise dopaminergic neurons elsewhere in the CNS and periphery, giving rise to many unwanted side-effects, e.g. serious disturbances of movement as a result of their adverse effects on the dopamine neurons involved in Parkinsonism (*see* Chapter 14). The diagnosis of schizophrenia should be reached cautiously – it requires far more than the presence of hallucinations, which can have many causes, including many drugs. The diagnosis should always be made by a specialist, as should the treatment plan, which should include prolonged courses of supportive psychotherapy, as well as appropriate maintenance drug treatment.

Drug treatment of schizophrenia

The treatment of schizophrenia is not restricted to drug interventions, which should always be supported by psychological and social interventions, carefully planned for the individual patient.

Drug classification of antipsychotics is about as vague as a classification could be! It amounts to 'old drugs' and 'new drugs', usually referred to as 'classical/typical' and 'atypical'. It is an honest reflection of our ignorance! However, they are all highly effective and they all strongly antagonise dopamine receptors in the brain amygdala.

The 'classical' group are subdivided into five groups, the members of each being chemically similar. These are:

1   the phenothiazines (e.g. fluphenazine)
2   the butyrophenones (e.g. haloperidol)
3   the diphenylbutylpiperidines (e.g. pimozide)
4   the thioxanthenes (e.g. flupentixol)
5   the substituted benzamides (e.g. sulpiride).

Do not worry about this terminology!

The clinical point is that different patients will do better with different chemical groups, as they find that one group controls their symptoms best or has fewer unpleasant side-effects, e.g. a drug may be selected because of its more sedative properties. As any psychiatrist will tell you, there is nothing linear (standardised) about human beings!

What are the advantages of the newer 'atypical' antipsychotics?

To understand that, one must realise that schizophrenia has 'positive' and 'negative' symptoms. The positive symptoms are delusions, hallucinations, thought disorder, and abnormal, stereotyped or aggressive behaviour, lasting at least six months. The classical antipsychotics control these to some degree in many patients. The atypical antipsychotics are no more effective in treating positive symptoms but are better tolerated because of their lower tendency to cause distressing neuromuscular side-effects.

The negative symptoms include social withdrawal and loss of feelings for others and oneself – 'flattened emotion'. These are more common in chronic schizophrenics, where the original negative symptoms may be supplemented by negativity as a side-effect of prolonged drug treatment and depression, and chronic institutionalisation. The atypical antipsychotics sometimes improve these symptoms, which are just as distressing to the patient and friends as the positive ones. Frequently used 'atypical' antipsychotic drugs are olanzapine, risperidone and quetiapine. See the *BNF* for the many caveats in antipsychotic drug treatment.

Side-effects of the antipsychotics

These are many, severe and some irreversible. The *BNF* briefly details most of them. To integrate with the rest of this section on drugs in the CNS, it is worth mentioning some side-effects which we could predict from knowledge gained in this book.

For example, Chapter 14, on Parkinson's disease, explained that the motor deficit there was due to lack of dopamine in one of the motor regulation centres (the substantia nigra) leading to interference with voluntary movement. Since all of the antipsychotics strongly antagonise dopamine receptors, it is predictable that Parkinson-like abnormalities of movement might follow its use, and that turns out to be one of the most serious and unpleasant side-effects of antipsychotic treatment, the 'extra-pyramidal' symptoms. They include Parkinsonian symptoms such as abnormal face and body movements, excessive muscle tone, restlessness and distressing repetitive involuntary movements of the tongue, jaw and face. They probably arise from disruption of the movement control system shown in Figure 14.1.

Psychosis is a vast clinical topic which has occupied the working lifetimes of many doctors and nurses. It is hoped that this chapter has given enough background to act as a starting point for those who have to prescribe or give antipsychotic medicines. As always, the *BNF* remains the authority on all aspects of prescribing – choice, dosage, cautions, contraindications, side-effects and interactions. But if in doubt regarding antipsychotic treatment, it is best always to refer to the supervising specialist.

Key points

- The dopamine–glutamate theory as to the biochemical pathology of schizophrenia is briefly described.
- The drug options in managing schizophrenia are listed, to be combined always with supportive psychotherapy.
- The 'positive' and 'negative' symptoms of chronic schizophrenia are described.
- The advantages of the newer antipsychotic drugs are described.
- The many serious side-effects of all these drugs are outlined.

18 Antidepressant drugs

Depression is a disorder of mood, varying from a mild normal reaction to life's vicissitudes, requiring a sympathetic ear, through moderate depression which may respond best to brief psychotherapy, to severe, clinical depression with a strong risk of suicide. The latter requires a determined management plan, including an effective antidepressant drug and regular psychotherapy. The symptoms must have been present for at least a month and should preferably include at least four of the following, elicited by a careful mental state examination, before a diagnosis is made and treatment is considered:

1 low mood, loss of happiness or equanimity, loss of hope
2 mood not improved by pleasant events or relationships
3 loss of enjoyment of everyday life
4 loss of interest in things and people
5 sleep disturbance, varying from insomnia to spending most of the day in bed
6 difficulty in concentrating and making decisions
7 withdrawal from personal relationships
8 slowing of thought processes and physical activity.

When should antidepressant drugs be prescribed?

Antidepressants are of little value in acute or mild depression, where brief psychotherapy is often very effective. They are effective in moderate depression, though psychotherapy is equally effective. Antidepressants are clearly indicated in severe depression, where psychotherapy and drug treatment are complementary, each increasing the effect of the other. Note that all antidepressant drugs have at least twenty lines of adverse side-effect listed in the *BNF*.

If little is known of the pharmacology of antipsychotic drugs (Chapter 17), still less is known about the CNS actions of the antidepressants. There are three groups of classical (typical) antidepressant:

1   the tricyclic antidepressants (e.g. amitriptyline) – the TCAs
2   the selective serotonin reuptake inhibitors (e.g. fluoxetine (Prozac)) – the SSRIs
3   the reversible monoamine oxidase-A inhibitor (RIMA) (e.g. moclobemide).

They all relieve severe depression in a large proportion of patients. Some patients respond very much better to one group than another. Groups 1 and 2 can be initiated relatively safely in primary care (given the diagnostic criteria above), but because of its extra risks, the RIMA should be started by a specialist. To maintain remission, drug treatment should be continued for six months, though some recurrently depressed patients may need prolonged treatment. It is not uncommon for depression to be associated with anxiety, termed 'agitated depression'. Such patients often do best on the older TCAs, which have marked sedative properties. SSRIs are much less sedating, but they have many other side-effects (*see* the *BNF*). Well-tried rating scales may be used to assess improvement in patients undergoing treatment, e.g. the Hamilton Rating Scale, or the newer Montgomery–Asberg Scale.

What is known about the action of antidepressants in the brain?

Because all effective antidepressants have been shown in animal experiments to increase the availability of the monoamines noradrenaline or serotonin (5-HT) or both, in the CNS, the only theory we have is that depression is caused by a 'functional deficit' of these neurotransmitters. The only additional 'hard' information is that TCAs and SSRIs block the reuptake of the neurotransmitter from its synapse (*see* Chapter 11, Figure 11.1), making more of it available for inter-nerve signalling. The TCAs and the SSRIs both block reuptake of noradrenaline and serotonin, but the SSRIs are very selective for serotonin reuptake and some more modern TCAs are very selective for noradrenaline reuptake (e.g. reboxetine).

The RIMA moclobemide acts by blocking the enzyme which metabolises (breaks down) the monoamines serotonin and noradrenaline, MAO-A. Reducing its breakdown in the pre-synaptic neuron and the cells around the synapse (glial cells) makes a greater concentration of the neurotransmitter available. For some reason, moclobemide improves mood within a few days, compared to the 3–4 week latent period of TCAs and SSRIs, but some dietary precautions limit its prescribing to specialists. *Patients on moclobemide must not be given an opioid analgesic, particularly pethidine.*

Manic-depressive (bipolar) illness

Some patients have a cyclical illness, with mood swinging from periods of extreme euphoria to periods of severe (often suicidal) depression. Such patients require assessment and prolonged regular follow-up by a specialist psychiatric unit. Oral lithium salts are still the first-line prophylactic (preventive) treatment in most patients. In bipolar illness, lithium acts as a 'mood stabiliser', i.e. it reduces the amplitude (extent) of mood swings, removing the extreme euphoria and the severity of depression. How it does this is still unknown, despite our good knowledge of its biochemical effects at the cellular level.

Lithium is a very risky drug, with a narrow therapeutic index, i.e. there is only a small difference between the plasma lithium concentration which is effective and that which is progressively toxic. See the *BNF*, section 4.2.3, for the signs of lithium toxicity, which can cause kidney damage, coma, convulsions and death. Monthly serum lithium monitoring is mandatory.

Second-line treatments of bipolar illness include carbamazepine and valproate, which act as 'mood stabilisers', whose true CNS actions are also unknown.

Key points

- The importance of diagnosis of depression and assessment of its severity are stressed.
- Antidepressant drugs are valuable in severe depression but no better than psychotherapy in mild or moderate depression.
- The monoamine theory of depression is mentioned.
- The main effective antidepressant drugs are described – the tricyclics (TCA), the selective serotonin reuptake inhibitors (SSRI), the reversible monoamine oxidase-A inhibitor (RIMA).
- The value and risks of lithium treatment of bipolar (manic-depressive) illness are covered.

19 Anti-epileptic drugs

Epilepsy is common and, in the absence of drug treatment, can be very disabling. It consists of unpredictable seizures in which abnormal 'showers' of neuronal discharge occur in one brain area, which may or may not spread across the brain. Seizures range from a few seconds' 'absence'* or loss of attention, to a convulsive fit lasting several minutes and threatening life itself by preventing respiration. All new cases of epilepsy should be referred to a specialist, whose access to a battery of tests is essential for diagnosis and management plan – see below.

All anti-epileptic drugs act by reducing the excitability of neurons throughout the brain. In convulsive fits ('grand mal epilepsy'*), intravenous lorazepam is given slowly to depolarise all GABA$_A$-controlled chloride ion channels (*see* Chapter 13) throughout the brain. A medical emergency.

This drug is unsuitable for the prevention of epilepsy, for like all benzodiazepines, it is very sedative and incompatible with normal life, and tolerance develops quickly (*see* Chapter 20). For prevention, we need drugs which preferentially block neurons firing at high frequency but which do not much affect other neurons, i.e. they allow normal thought, concentration and all activity to proceed, but block the sorts of intense neuronal discharges involved in an epileptic seizure. Several drugs have been found whose action can be explained on that basis. For preventing convulsive seizures the drugs carbamazepine, phenytoin, valproate and lamotrigine are well established and usually well tolerated. The earliest successful anti-epileptic, still in occasional use, is phenobarbitone (a barbiturate), which also potentiates GABA$_A$-gated Cl$^-$ channels, like the benzodiazepines, and is consequently somewhat sedative. Ten newer anti-epileptic drugs are now available. Their use should be led by a consultant neurologist – see *BNF*, section 4.8.1. As far as is known, all anti-epileptic drugs act at one or more of the following three ion channels: (a) GABA-gated Cl$^-$ ion channels, enhancing the inhibitory effect of GABA, e.g. lorazepam for severe fits; (b) Na$^+$ channels, blocking preferentially intensive neuronal activity (use dependence), e.g. carbamazepine, lamotrigine, phenobarbitone; (c) T-type Ca^{++} channels in the CNS, e.g. ethosuximide, valproate, clonazepam.

---

* Such French terms as 'absence', 'petit mal' and 'grand mal' show recognition of the pre-eminence of French physicians in early neurology and psychiatry.

For 'absence' seizures ('petit mal epilepsy'*) valproate or ethosuximide are the drugs of choice.

The management of epilepsy is a life-long duty and should be undertaken as 'shared care', with regular review by a specialist. The *BNF*, as always, has short informative paragraphs on all the anti-epileptic drugs.

Aetiology (causes) of epilepsy

These are:

- unknown or idiopathic (the commonest)
- head injury
- tumours
- meningitis and encephalitis
- ischaemia
- diabetic crises (hypo- or hyperglycaemic)
- withdrawal from alcohol or drugs
- degenerative disease of the brain, e.g. Alzheimer's
- syphilis.

It is the neurologist's job to exclude the last eight on this list before making a firm diagnosis of idiopathic epilepsy.

The importance of the patient's compliance/adherence in self-medication

Abrupt cessation of preventive treatment risks severe rebound fits (seizures), even when the patient has been free from symptoms for years. Research has shown that about 20% of all patients comply very well with their medication, 40% comply well enough to derive benefit, while 40% comply very poorly, including 15% who rarely have their prescriptions dispensed; *see* Chapter 30.

Key points

- The neuronal basis of epilepsy is described.
- The drug treatment of convulsive epileptic fits is described.
- The very different drugs needed to prevent epilepsy (prophylaxis) are described.
- The aetiology of epilepsy (its origins) are listed.

---

20 Drugs of abuse: hallucinogens and CNS stimulants

All clinicians – doctors, nurses and paramedics – should have a basic understanding of drugs of abuse, since their use is now so widespread in all sections of society and their presentation as emergencies is now so common. As in many drugs affecting the CNS we know their pharmacology in animal models, we know their gross CNS effects in humans and we speculate as to cause and effect. If we group these drugs according to their observed effects we have:

1 the CNS stimulants – the amphetamines (including ecstasy), cocaine and 'crack-cocaine'
2 the hallucinogens (in jargon, the psychotomimetics) – LSD and cannabis
3 opioids – morphine and particularly diamorphine (heroin) and codeine
4 CNS depressants – alcohol, solvents, barbiturates and the benzodiazepines
5 tobacco/nicotine.

Some people will try anything! Worse than that (for the casualty nurse or doctor on call) they will often take a 'cocktail' of drugs from any of groups 1–5. Bear that in mind – it may save an addict's life.

What is addiction?

'Recreational' drugs are all taken for their pleasant, euphoriant effects which stimulate the 'reward' mechanisms in the brain to reinforce behaviour. Therein lies their tendency to cause addiction. Pleasurable experience leads to repetition of the drug-taking (*habituation*). As the brain counters the drug effect by up-regulation or down-regulation of the specific receptors (*see* Chapter 7), the user needs to take larger doses of the drug (*tolerance*). Eventually, the user becomes dependent on the drug, psychologically and often physically – *dependence*, with a craving for the drug and very unpleasant withdrawal effects if the craving is not satisfied ('cold turkey'). With the passage of time, the drug of dependence becomes central to the patient's life, often at a cost to their occupational, social and family lives. There may be substantial adverse physical and psychological effects. This poses a formidable challenge for clinicians working in addiction centres, who often have to use substitute drugs to ease the patient's misery, provide sterile hypodermic syringes and needles and encourage their patients' continuation in therapy. Substitute prescribing minimises harm to addicts from impure and unpredictable illicit drugs and reduces secondary damage due to criminal and risk-taking behaviour. 'Main-lining' (intravenous self-injection) using shared needles risks infection with the AIDS virus and/or hepatitis C.

CNS stimulants (amphetamines and cocaine)

All of these act by releasing large quantities of the catecholamines dopamine and noradrenaline from brain nuclei or by preventing their physiological breakdown. They are rapidly very addictive, and repeated use often gives rise to behaviours mimicking schizophrenia (drug-induced psychoses). Neural tolerance rapidly occurs and larger and larger doses are needed to achieve the desired euphoric 'hit'. Personality changes soon become apparent to those who know the users best.

On the positive side, the CNS stimulants methylphenidate (Ritalin) and modafinil (Provigil) are well-established specialist treatments. Methylphenidate is of proven value in attention deficit hyperactivity disorder (ADHD) and modafinil is of great benefit in managing the sudden 'sleep attacks' of narcolepsy. *See* Table 20.1.

The related CNS stimulant fenfluramine should not be used as an appetite suppressant (*see BNF*, section 4.5.2).

The hallucinogens

LSD (lysergic acid diethylamide) acts as a very potent agonist at serotonin (5-HT$_2$) brain receptors, producing hallucinations and delusions, many of them pleasant ('psychedelic'), but quite often terrifying ('a bad trip'). As with the CNS stimulants, frequent use often leads to prolonged psychotic periods. Yet LSD is not considered dependence producing.

Cannabis appears to act on specific 'cannabinoid' receptors in brain centres thought to be associated with memory, aversion/reward and motor (movement) control. It is used to achieve increased sensory experience, relaxation and euphoria. It is less addictive than the opiates, tobacco or alcohol, but long-term use is now thought to cause psychosis (hospital clinicians admitting a psychotic young person ask first if he/she is a regular cannabis user), and serious deterioration of personality – a terrible price to pay.

Cannabinoids are being investigated as possible adjunctive (add-on) therapy of intractable neuropathic pain and for prevention of nausea in palliative care. Tetrahydrocannabinol (Sativex) is now licensed for specialist use in the UK. It has proved effective in treating aspects of multiple sclerosis.

The opioids

The most important (and on the street, expensive) of these is, of course, heroin (diamorphine). The pharmacology of these drugs has been briefly described in Chapter 15. Heroin gives users a 'wonderful' euphoria – peace, contentment and relaxation (part of its great clinical value in injury and terminal care). The maximum effect (the 'rush') is achieved by intravenous self-injection, exposing the user to the risks of AIDS, hepatitis B and C and other diseases transferred in blood by needle-sharing. Tolerance, dependence and addiction occur rapidly, after which users' lives may be entirely occupied with getting the next 'fix', leading to petty crime and prostitution. Heroin addicts often raid GPs' surgeries and pharmacies and may forge prescriptions if they can get the blank NHS prescription forms. Keep yours locked up! Withdrawal is severe and rehabilitation is prolonged and often unsuccessful. Heroin addiction is among the hardest to treat; patients may need long periods of substitution therapy with daily methadone, in the context of a multidisciplinary team approach. *See* Table 20.1.

CNS depressants

Alcohol and solvents are cell poisons, damaging many tissues, particularly the liver, which has the task of detoxifying them (metabolism – *see* Chapters 3 and 4). Recent research suggests that alcohol has a benzodiazepine-like effect (*see* Chapter 13), and that it may inhibit glutamate receptors (*see* Chapter 11, Table 11.1). Its metabolism is sluggish so that it rapidly accumulates after the first few drinks (*see* Chapter 3). It is, of course, very addictive in a proportion of the population. Alcohol is responsible for ten times more chronic illness, personality deterioration, social disruption and death than any of the more recent 'recreational' drugs, though that statistic may be due to its much more widespread and legal use. It is also responsible for much antisocial behaviour and the breakdown of relationships.

Tobacco/nicotine

This is one of the most seriously addictive drugs of all, responsible for a large proportion of premature heart and artery disease and death, for almost all chronic bronchitis and a large proportion of lung, oesophageal, bladder and pancreatic cancers. It causes excitation of nicotinic acetylcholine receptors in the brain and periphery. Tobacco addicts have been subclassified as (a) peak seekers and (b) trough avoiders, the latter tending to be chain-smokers attempting to maintain their brain concentration of nicotine. About 5% of nicotine addicts manage to 'quit'. Dermal nicotine patches or chewing gum help some people and avoid many of the risks of tobacco smoke.

Table 20.1 Neurotransmitters, drugs affecting them, known effects of these drugs and diseases treated by them.

Neurotransmitter (alternative name)	Receptor type	Drug group(s) affecting	Example drug(s)	Known effects of drug	Disease(s) treated
Noradrenaline (Norepinephrine)	Noradrenergic and serotonergic (non-selective)	Tricyclic antidepressants (TCAs)	amitriptyline	Effective antidepressant: augments effects of noradrenaline and serotonin by blocking reuptake	Depression and agitated depression (has a sedative effect)
Serotonin (5-hydroxytryptamine, 5-HT)	Serotonergic (5-HT) selective	Selective serotonin reuptake inhibitors (SSRIs)	fluoxetine (Prozac)	Effective antidepressant; augments effects of serotonin	Depression (less sedating than TCAs)
	Serotonergic ($5-HT_3$) in CNS	'Setron' anti-emetics – $5-HT_3$ antagonists	ondansetron	Powerful anti-emetic. Blocks $5-HT_3$ receptors in chemoreceptor trigger zone (CTZ) in CNS	Extreme nausea and vomiting, e.g. in cancer chemotherapy
	Serotonergic ($5-HT_4$) in intestine	Gastro-intestinal $5-HT_4$ receptor agonists	metoclopramide	Stimulates peristalsis-controlled gastro-intestinal propulsion	Non-ulcer dyspepsia and gastro-oesophageal reflux (GORD)
	Serotonergic ($5-HT_{1A}$)	CNS $5-HT_{1A}$ partial agonist	buspirone	Delayed-action anxiolytic	Specialist management of anxiety
	Serotonergic ($5-HT_{1D}$)	CNS $5-HT_{1D}$ agonists – the 'triptans'	sumatriptan	Vasoconstriction of arteries throughout the body – may precipitate angina	Acute migraine and 'cluster' headaches
	Serotonergic ($5-HT_1$)	Ergotamine group (alkaloids) $5-HT_1$ antagonists	ergotamine	Vasoconstriction of arteries throughout the body. Also raises BP by stimulating alpha-adrenoceptors – a risky drug	Specialist management of migraine and 'cluster' headache prophylaxis (prevention)
Dopamine	Dopaminergic D_2	All antipsychotic drugs	flupentixol olanzapine	Antagonise excess dopamine release from amygdala and other CNS centres	Schizophrenia – remove many symptoms and sedate without impairing consciousness
	Dopamine, noradrenaline and serotonin receptors	All amphetamines and related drugs are highly unselective agonists at all these receptors	*dexamphetamine *MDMA *cocaine	Cause intense release of dopamine, noradrenaline and serotonin in CNS and inhibit their reuptake	Strongly-addictive 'recreational' drugs
			methylphenidate (Ritalin)	Unknown mode of action	Attention deficit/hyperactivity disorder in children – specialist use
			fenfluramine	As for dexamphetamine	Appetite suppressant – not in BNF

(continued)

Neurotransmitter (alternative name)	Receptor type	Drug group(s) affecting	Example drug(s)	Known effects of drug	Disease(s) treated
Dopamine (cont.)	Dopaminergic D$_2$ receptors in CTZ	Dopamine D$_2$ receptor antagonists	metoclopramide and domperidone	Block dopamine D$_2$ receptors in chemoreceptor trigger zone (CTZ) – see Chapter 16	Powerful anti-emetics and gastro-intestinal peristaltic stimulants – see serotonergic action above
	Dopaminergic neurons in substantia nigra of CNS	Levodopa, given always with a dopa-decarboxylase inhibitor (see Chapter 14)	co-careldopa co-beneldopa	Replenish dopamine deficit in movement regulation centre of CNS	The mainstay of treatment of Parkinsonism
Opioid peptides	μ (mu) opioid receptors	All morphine-like (opioid) mu-receptor agonists in the CNS; also act at spinal cord level (suppressing upward transmission of pain stimuli)	*morphine *diamorphine *methadone fentanyl, etc . . .	Cause hyperpolarisation of pain centre neurons, thus inhibiting release of their pain-sensation impulses to higher centres – see Chapter 15. Also act in spinal cord, suppressing upward transmission of pain stimuli to brain	The most powerful analgesics known. Also have a beneficial euphoric effect, e.g. in terminal disease. Often cause severe nausea and severe respiratory and cardiac depression. All are very addictive
	μ (mu) opioid receptors	Opioid antagonist	naloxone	Displaces all opiates from the mu receptors throughout the body and so reverses all opiate effects	Opiate overdosage, given intravenously. Highly effective and life-saving, but has a much shorter half-life than the opiates and must be repeated if signs of opioid overdose recur
Glutamate	**NMDA ion channel	NMDA channel blockers	*ketamine	Blocks fast excitatory neuronal transmission in CNS	Short-acting intravenous anaesthetic, useful in children. May cause post-anaesthetic psychotic symptoms – hallucinations.
			memantine	Blocks fast excitatory neuronal transmission in CNS	Reduction of brain damage after stroke and head injury. Modest cognitive improvement in moderate and severe Alzheimer's disease
GABA (gamma-aminobutyric acid)	GABA$_A$	All benzodiazepines	*diazepam temazepam midazolam	Sedative Hypnotic Deep sedation	Anxiety Insomnia Day procedure anaesthetic
		Benzodiazepine antagonist	flumazenil	Benzodiazepine antagonist	Benzodiazepine overdose

* Asterisks denote drugs of abuse.
**NMDA = N-methyl-D-aspartate

Summary

It may be constructive for the reader who has completed Chapters 11–19 to revisit Table 20.1 which at the outset of study may have appeared overwhelming, but which should now be an easily understood summary of what is known about drugs in the CNS.

Key points

- The 'steps' of addiction are described.
- The different classes of drugs of abuse are listed.
- What is known about each class's action on the brain is described.

---

21 Alzheimer's disease

Dementia is the progressive impairment of intellectual functions with loss of several cognitive (thinking) abilities, of which the most striking is usually memory loss and, later, loss of the ability to speak coherently, understand the speech of others or perform simple daily tasks. Alzheimer's disease (AD) is dementia without a known cause such as stroke, alcoholism or brain trauma. At the age of 65, AD affects 5% of people, at age 95, 90%. About two-thirds of dementia will prove to be Alzheimer's disease.

Recent research shows that many neurodegenerative diseases, including AD, begin with the 'misfolding' and aggregation of certain intracellular proteins. If these abnormal proteins are not removed by the neuron's defence mechanisms, aggregation leads to large complexes such as amyloid plaques and neurofibrillary tangles, with resulting death of neurons.

There are three major neuro-chemical malfunctions in AD, each of them contributing to accelerated nerve cell death:

1 excessive neuronal stimulation by the excitatory neurotransmitter glutamate
2 deficit of the protective neuronal growth factors
3 loss of biochemical defence against attack by reactive oxygen species (oxidative stress).

No drugs are yet available to counter the progression of any of these, though epidemiological studies have associated simple NSAIDs like ibuprofen with reduced risk of AD.

On a brighter note, research has also shown that AD sufferers have a loss of cholinergic neuronal function due to reduced ability both to synthesise acetyl choline (ACh) and to recycle it for reuse. The drugs donepezil, rivastigmine and galantamine all reduce the metabolism (breakdown) of ACh, while memantine blocks glutamate transmission. They all give a slight improvement in memory, thought and quality of life, but are effective in less than 50% of patients. They may all cause a variety of unpleasant adverse drug reactions, some severe. The *BNF* stresses that these drugs 'should be initiated and supervised only by a specialist experienced in the management of dementia'. Their use should cease if there is no measurable improvement after three months' treatment. About half of responders may show a slowing of the rate of progress of AD, but nothing known at present will stop it.

While treatment should be started by a dementia specialist, care may be effectively shared by the primary care team, but the stress on caregivers cannot be overemphasised.

Key points

■ The signs of dementia are described.

■ The three known neuro-chemical abnormalities of Alzheimer's disease are listed.

■ The limited drug interventions are described.

DRUG TOPICS OF SPECIAL IMPORTANCE

22 How the many antidiabetic drugs work

Introduction

Glucose is the main source of energy for all body cells. Except in starvation, glucose is derived from digested food. Since food intake is intermittent, glucose becomes available in surges which require strict regulation to maintain plasma glucose within the normal range of 60–110 mg/dL (3.1–6.1 mmol/L).

There is no more complex physiology than that of glucose regulation, involving intestinal hormones, hormones from the A, B and D cells of the pancreatic islets of Langerhans, chemical messengers in liver cells and an array of glucose transporters in most cell membranes. Fortunately, a detailed knowledge of this physiology is not essential to understand how current antidiabetic drugs work, for they act on a limited number of effector sites.

Diabetes mellitus – Type 1 and Type 2

Type 1 diabetes may occur at any age and involves complete loss of insulin secretion due to pancreatic B cell destruction usually by an autoimmune process. Untreated, this causes profound metabolic disruption and illness due to ketoacidosis with dehydration, gross plasma electrolyte disturbance, coma and death. The only treatments of Type 1 diabetes are insulin injections and diet.

Type 2 diabetes occurs predominantly in the over-40 age group and in people with abdominal obesity. In Type 2, insulin secretion is initially normal or above-normal but the peripheral tissues have become relatively insensitive to insulin ('insulin resistance'). The B cells at first enlarge (hypertrophy), then slowly fail. Type 2 diabetes is successfully treated by diet, oral drugs and exercise, but over time the B cell failure is complete and insulin must be added to preserve health. How these oral drugs work is the main subject of this chapter.

Clinicians participating in diabetic care – doctors, specialist nurses and pharmacists

– need much more clinical knowledge than these short paragraphs, and any medical text will supply this. At the introductory level, the account of diabetes in *Treating Common Diseases*, may be useful.[1]

Treating Type 1 diabetes

Treatment should always be initiated and reviewed by a specialist team – physician, dietitian and nurse. Care can then be shared with the community team – GP, specialist nurse, pharmacist. The treatment always involves the regular subcutaneous injection of insulin, life-long. The drug industry has provided us with a range of short-acting, medium-acting and long-acting insulins which, with good co-operation by the patient, can mimic the body's natural insulin secretion pattern with minimal disruption of the patient's lifestyle. These insulins are succinctly described in the *British National Formulary* (*BNF*), Chapter 6.1.1.

The other essential element of Type 1 diabetic treatment is diet, which is also a life-long requirement. Regular review by a dietitian helps to keep the patient compliant. The most skilful patients learn to 'calorie count' so as to adjust their insulin dose according to the carbohydrate content of a meal.

How insulin works

Most body cells, but particularly those of the liver, muscle and fatty (adipose) tissue, have specific insulin receptors on their cell membranes. Insulin binding to its receptor stimulates a cascade of metabolic events within the cell. Depending on the tissue and the receptor, those events include the uptake and storage of glucose, fats and amino acids after a meal. Excess glucose is stored as glycogen and fat, and amino acids are stored as protein – all stimulated by insulin binding to specific receptors in different tissues. On the longer term, insulin stimulates cell growth and development from foetal growth to adult repair and replacement. Insulin is the major hormone governing metabolism (in combination with the complex array of control processes which research has revealed, and beyond the scope of this basic textbook).

Treating Type 2 diabetes

1 Drugs which stimulate insulin-release from the failing B cells.
Several commonly prescribed oral antidiabetic drugs act along the pathway by which raised plasma glucose causes insulin release. It is not difficult to understand. Please study Figure 22.1, together with its commentary, following the sequence 1–8.

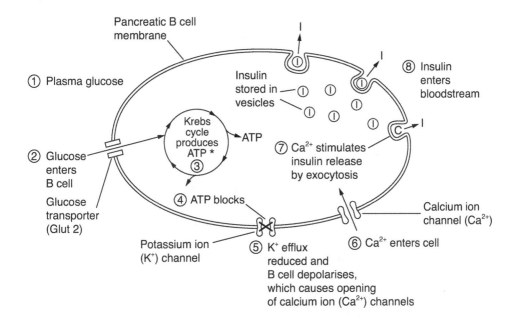

Figure 22.1 Simplified diagram of pancreatic B cell, showing how glucose entering the cell causes insulin release into the bloodstream. * The Krebs cycle (tricarboxylic acid cycle) is the 'final pathway' of oxidative energy release from carbohydrates, fats and proteins, trapping energy as ATP – adenosine triphosphate, to power metabolism.

① Plasma glucose concentration rises (the major stimulant of insulin release). This rise is sensed by glucose transporters in the B cell membrane, so-called 'Glut 2'.
② Glucose enters the cell, is phosphorylated and enters the Krebs cycle.
③ The Krebs cycle produces molecules of adenosine triphosphate (ATP).
④ ATP blocks the ATP-sensitive potassium channels, which reduces ⑤ K^+ ion efflux from the cell. That causes depolarisation of the cell.
⑥ As a result of depolarisation, voltage-dependent calcium channels open (*see* Chapter 9) and Ca^{2+} enters the B cell – calcium influx.
⑦ Ca^{2+} stimulates the release of pre-formed insulin from storage vesicles, by exocytosis.
⑧ Insulin enters the bloodstream via porous (fenestrated) capillaries surrounding the B cells.

Studying Figure 22.1 allows us immediate understanding of the action of several commonly prescribed oral antidiabetic drugs, which all act at step 4. Blockage of the K^+ channels leads to steps 5 to 8, releasing more insulin from the failing B cells' vesicles. These drugs are:

1 *The sulfonylureas* gliclazide, glipizide, glimepiride and tolbutamide.
2 *The meglitinides* repaglinide and nateglinide.

N.B. As Type 2 diabetes deteriorates, one or more antidiabetic drugs with different glucose-lowering actions can be added (see below).

In due course, the B cells fail completely and the Type 2 diabetic requires subcutaneous insulin from then on.

It cannot be overstressed that strict diet is as essential in good Type 2 management as in Type 1. Regular, rhythmic exercise is beneficial in both types. Insulin-sensitive tissue (muscle, liver and adipose tissue) have special glucose transporters (Glut 4) which actively transport glucose into the cell (independently of insulin) in response to exercise.

How the other oral antidiabetic drugs work

The remaining oral antidiabetics do not act on B cells but reduce plasma glucose by a number of other actions. Everyone involved in treating Type 2 diabetic patients should understand all of these, and how and why they can be combined with the sulfonylureas and meglitinides (see above).

1 *Metformin.* This is one of the most frequently prescribed oral antidiabetics. It reduces plasma glucose first, by reducing glucose synthesis in the liver; second, by increasing insulin action in fat and muscle; and third, by reducing glucose absorption from the intestine. It will not work unless the patient's B cells are secreting some insulin. Metformin is the drug of first choice in obese Type 2 diabetes, and as the condition deteriorates, it can be combined with all of the oral antidiabetic drugs mentioned above and below, and with insulin when that is needed. It has some side-effects and should not be used in patients with renal, or hepatic or cardiac failure or in advanced chronic obstructive pulmonary disease (COPD).

2 *Pioglitazone.* One of the features of Type 2 diabetes is tissue insensitivity to insulin, often called 'insulin resistance'. This involves particularly liver, muscle and fat. Insulin resistance is strongly associated with abdominal obesity. Pioglitazone reduces peripheral insulin resistance, thus 'making the most' of the remaining insulin. It also reduces glucose output by the liver. It is often combined with metformin and/or a sulfonylurea.

3 *The gliptins.* Linagliptin, saxagliptin, sitagliptin and vildagliptin act in the mucous membrane of the duodenum and small intestine, causing release of peptide hormones which slow the rate of gastric emptying, reduce pancreatic glucagon secretion (A cells) and begin insulin secretion in 'anticipation' of the rise in plasma glucose which results from the meal.

4 *Exenatide.* This drug must be taken by subcutaneous injection. It mimics the effects of one of the intestinal peptide hormones (*see* 3 above), with similar therapeutic results. It also reduces appetite, helping weight loss. Liraglutide and lixisenatide have similar actions and must also be injected subcutaneously.

5 *Acarbose.* By delaying carbohydrate absorption, acarbose lowers the 'peak' of plasma

glucose following a meal. Patients often dislike its side-effects (intestinal), well-described in *BNF*, Chapter 6.1.2.

6 *Dapagliflozin*. This new drug reduces glucose reabsorption from the renal tubule (*see* Chapter 4), increasing urinary glucose excretion. Dapagliflozin is ineffective in even moderate renal failure.

Comment

The thoughtful reader should now understand how a skilled diabetic specialist can tailor a patient's Type 2 medication using up to three different oral hypoglycaemic (glucose-lowering) drugs, so as to obtain an optimal control of plasma glucose and so minimise the terrible complications of poorly controlled diabetes – irreversible damage to eyes, kidneys, arterioles, heart, skin and nervous system. Reason: the ability to use drugs whose functions are different, but complementary.

Glucagon. This is an important hormone secreted by the A cells of the pancreatic islets. Its secretion is stimulated by a fall in plasma glucose concentration. In the liver it promotes rapid glucose production by stimulating the breakdown of liver glycogen. Its other functions are complex and beyond the scope of this book.

Use. In hypoglycaemic coma (loss of consciousness due to low plasma glucose), the best treatment is the intravenous injection of 20% glucose solution. If that is not possible, glucagon can be injected subcutaneously or intra-muscularly. That makes possible its lifesaving use by emergency nurses and paramedics.

Reference

1 McGavock H and Johnston GD (2007) *Treating Common Diseases*. Radcliffe Publishing, Oxford, New York.

23 Treating severe chronic inflammation

For many years, clinicians have struggled to achieve symptomatic relief, let alone cure, of several diseases in which the primary cause is uncontrolled inflammation in body tissues, particularly rheumatoid arthritis (RA) and inflammatory bowel disease (IBD), either Crohn's disease or ulcerative colitis.

The body's powerful immune system is its white blood cells, of which 2–3% are circulating in the blood. The remainder are located in the lymph nodes and spleen. These, in good health, provide a powerful defence against foreign protein invasion and other tissue damage, including viral, bacterial and parasitic infections. They also recognise most cancerous cells as foreign, and destroy them. The immune system is highly sophisticated and specific – it produces exactly the level of response needed, tailored specifically to each individual threat.

In RA and IBD, however, the immune system attacks some of the body's normal tissues as though they were foreign protein. What's more, the level of inflammatory response is out of control, destroying the joints (RA) or colonic mucosa (IBD). And in RA at least, many other body tissues may be attacked, though to a lesser degree – it is a systemic disease.

These diseases are progressive, if untreated, and cause the severest symptoms, ruining the patient's quality of life, leading to great and prolonged disability and sometimes death.

Over the past 55 years, groups of drugs have been discovered which attenuate and even halt this 'rogue' inflammatory process. The actions of these drugs are partially understood in some cases. They involve some of the most complex pharmacology, well beyond the scope of this book.[1,2,3] These drugs are all risky and most are initiated by specialists in each field, but since primary care clinicians often share the ongoing care, it is important that readers should have a basic knowledge of them and a general concept of their actions. Please study Table 23.1 and Figure 23.1. Table 23.1 summarises (1) the main modern drugs used to manage RA and IBD, (2) their action in quelling the overactive immune system, and (3) the diseases in which they are at least partially successful. Note that at any given time, more than one of these drugs will be used. That is a fine clinical judgement, according to the response to treatment, or lack of it. Study Figure 23.1 and its commentary.

Table 23.1 is listed as (approximately), a 'therapeutic staircase', each downward step a

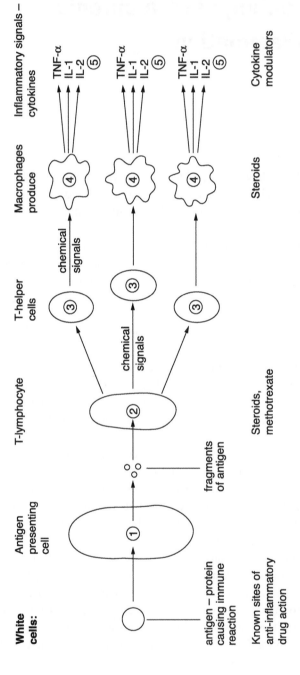

Figure 23.1 Part of the inflammatory process – *see text for commentary. Note that each group of white cells is highly specialised for its rôle in the process.*

progressively more powerful (and risky) intervention. The first entry (the steroids) are the exception: they are sometimes used early in the diseases, but can also be life-saving in severe recurrences. Their use is always for as short a period as possible because of their widespread metabolic effects.

Figure 23.1 is a very simplified account of the process by which the cytokines (chemical signals) which drive chronic inflammation are synthesised by the immune system's white cells. Note that each 'step' is the responsibility of a specialised family of white cells. Reading from left to right:

1   The large macrophages engulf foreign protein, the antigen (e.g. a bacterium or virus), and then 'present' fragments of it to . . .
2   a specialised T-lymphocyte, 'arming' it and causing it to secrete chemical signals which . . .
3   result in the proliferation of a further set of lymphocytes, the T-helper cells. T-helper cells stimulate proliferation of . . .
4   specialised macrophages which secrete the cytokines Interleukin 1 and 2 (IL-1, IL-2) and tumour necrosis factor-alpha (TNF-α). These, if unopposed by normal regulatory factors, lead to a 'forest fire' of inflammation in affected tissues, which until recently, has been very hard to control.
5   Figure 23.1 also indicates the stages in the inflammatory process at which modern anti-inflammatory drugs are thought to act.

For each inflammatory cytokine there is, in good health, an equally powerful anti-inflammatory cytokine (not shown, for clarity). Why these control signals fail in RA and IBD is not known.

In normal health, when the invading organism has been destroyed, yet further cytokines and other cell signals terminate the inflammatory response and promote repair of damaged tissue. Cell 'memory' of the antigen is retained by specialised white cells, which confer long-term immunity to that infection. They are the cause of 'auto-vaccination' and medicinal immunisation.

Table 23.1 Drugs used to manage rheumatoid arthritis and inflammatory bowel disease.

Drug	Action (numerals refer to Figure 23.1)	Disease
Steroids, e.g. prednisolone, budesonide (oral) triamcinolone (intra-articular injection)	Block the early propagation of inflammatory white cells (1). Deactivate inflammatory signals (cytokines) at the end of the process (4). *Note*: All oral steroids have serious side-effects and long-term oral use is to be avoided. Careful monitoring is essential – *see BNF*.	RA – often by injection into inflamed joints, to quell flare-ups. IBD – usually by local application to the lower colon in ulcerative colitis – foam enemas. Short-term oral use for severe flares of RA and IBD.
NSAIDs, e.g. ibuprofen, naproxen, diclofenac (oral)	Block the synthesis in tissues of inflammatory prostaglandins – *see Chapter 8*. Often used to ease pain and inflammation at the start of RA treatment, while DMARDs are taking effect. *Note*: All NSAIDs have many serious side-effects – *see Chapter 8 and BNF*.	RA – established place in early management. Osteoarthritis (OA) – in severe cases only and in low dosage.
DMARDs – disease-modifying anti-rheumatic drugs, e.g. methotrexate, mesalazine, azathioprine,	The mechanism of action of these drugs in RA and IBD is still unknown. They all 'quell' the immune response and they all have serious side-effects. Regular monitoring is a routine part of specialist care. *See BNF guidance*. *(DMARDs is a misnomer – these drugs are used for IBD and other rheumatic disease.)*	RA – methotrexate once weekly often the first choice. Takes up to 8 weeks to work. Often continued to maintain disease remission.

(continued)

Drug	Action (numerals refer to Figure 23.1)	Disease
leflunomide (oral)	Used when other DMARDs fail. Toxic. Has a very long half-life ($t_{1/2}$) – see Chapter 5.	IBD – both ulcerative colitis and Crohn's disease, usually starting with mesalazine, which is also the commonest maintenance therapy for ulcerative colitis. Azathioprine is often used for maintenance of remission in Crohn's disease.
Cytokine modulators, e.g. infliximab, adalimumab, etanercept (by injection)	All third-line treatment when DMARDs have failed. Block one of the strongest inflammatory signals to tissue cells – the cytokine TNF-α (tumour necrosis factor-alpha) – see (5) in Figure 23.1. Proved to suppress inflammation and slow down progression of joint destruction in RA. In Crohn's disease, produce complete remission in 33%, significant improvement in a further 33% but no response in the remaining third. Note: Because the cytokine modulators block an essential element in the immune process, they all risk serious infection of all types. They also have multiple unpleasant side-effects – see BNF.	Severe RA, sometimes in combination with a DMARD like methotrexate. Severe Crohn's disease – infliximab and adalimumab only. Ulcerative colitis – limited benefit. For severe UC, the only certain cure remains total colectomy.

Key points

- The normal function of the immune system is briefly described.
- Loss of control of the inflammatory response leads to chronic inflammation in one or more body tissues.
- A figure gives a simplified concept of the immune process.
- A table lists the main drugs used to treat chronic inflammation, with their actions.

References

1 Rang HP, Dale MM, Ritter JM and Flower RJ (2012) Local hormones, inflammation and immune reactions. In: *Rang and Dale's Pharmacology* (7e). Churchill Livingstone, Oxford.
2 Barrett KE, Barman SM, Boitano S *et al.* (2010) Immunity, infection and inflammation: In: *Ganong's Review of Medical Physiology* (23e). McGraw-Hill Medical, Columbus, OH.
3 Alberts B, Johnson A, Lewis J *et al.* (2008) The adaptive immune system. In: *Molecular Biology of the Cell* (5e). Garland Science, New York.

All good university libraries should hold a copy of these three books.

24 The scientific basis of prescribing for the elderly

Older people account for a growing percentage of the UK population, and for around one-third of primary care workload and prescribing volume. Unfortunately, several studies in European acute geriatric hospital departments have shown that 10–12% of all acute admissions of elderly patients and 18% of elderly deaths are the direct result of prescribed medicines.[1–3] This has been confirmed by a large American study in primary care.[4]

Drug:drug interaction is one of the commonest causes of these admissions, along with patient and carer confusion as to the dosage sequence of several concurrent medications. Such confusion may result in an excessively high dose, particularly of psychotropic drugs.

Hyperkalaemia* or hyponatraemia† may be caused by chronic diuretic therapy without proper monitoring of blood electrolytes. Build-up of plasma drug concentrations due to reduced liver and kidney function is common. One or more of the well-known side-effects and interactions of NSAIDs, which were considered in Chapter 8, are common causes of drug-associated illness in the elderly.

Box 24.1 summarises the problem and highlights that 27% of all adverse drug reactions (ADRs) reported to the Committee on Safety of Medicines (CSM) occur in the elderly; it also gives the underlying reasons for this prescribing phenomenon. Regular medication reviews of all elderly patients are essential.

The biological age of elderly patients

There is no such thing as a standard prescription for an elderly patient. Therefore it is important to assess the patient's biological age, i.e. is s/he a 'senior athlete' or chronically ill with multiple organ failure and pathology?

Common to all patients over the age of 70 are the physiological changes of ageing, leading to a gradual reduction in functional reserve in the cardiovascular, respiratory, renal, hepatic, musculoskeletal and central nervous systems, as well as the skin.

---

* hyperkalaemia = excessive plasma concentration of potassium
† hyponatraemia = low sodium concentration

Whether a patient's presenting symptoms are due to normal physiological ageing, requiring only reassurance, or to pathology requiring drug treatment, is often a difficult clinical judgement. Good geriatric care is pro-active–preventive.

Box 24.1 A large proportion of all adverse drug reactions (ADRs) occur in elderly patients, but these are vastly under-reported.

The problem
Over-65s account for:

- 33% of all prescriptions
- 27% of all reported ADRs; ratio female:male = 2:1
- 15% of population.

The reasons
Over-65s have:

- decreased salivation and swallowing, protein binding, drug metabolism/ elimination
- altered drug-tissue distribution and drug-tissue responses
- unavoidable polypharmacy (if multiple pathology is present)*
- poor medication compliance (often).

*e.g. it is not unusual for a 75-year-old to have hypertension, chronic heart failure, chronic kidney disease, diabetes and osteoarthritis, all requiring drug treatment.

Reduced drug metabolism and excretion

Tables 24.1–24.3 show the essential therapeutic considerations that every prescriber should check off whenever issuing or repeating a prescription for an older patient. The checklist consists of altered liver and kidney function, nutrition, tissue responses and body composition.

In Chapters 3 and 4 we considered drug metabolism and excretion, and Table 24.1 shows that decreased drug metabolism and excretion are normal in older patients, particularly those over the age of 70.

If standard adult doses of many drugs are given to this age group, excessive plasma concentrations will gradually accumulate. The problem is exacerbated by reduced kidney function and a resulting reduction in the ability to excrete drugs and their metabolites. The plasma half-lives of digoxin, lithium and gentamicin are doubled, while that of diazepam may be quadrupled.

The common prescription of NSAIDs for joint pain frequently accelerates this natural decline in renal function by inhibiting renal prostaglandin synthesis, causing tubular ischaemia and retention of sodium and water, which may, in turn, precipitate or worsen left ventricular (heart) failure.

Table 24.1 The normal ageing process – changes in liver and kidney function.

Liver changes	Kidney changes
• decreased blood flow leads to decreased presystemic drug metabolism • decreased liver size, microsomal (P450) oxidation and antipyrine clearances lead to decreased hepatic drug metabolism	• the number of nephrons decreases by 6% per decade; although serum creatinine may be normal, older people do have reduced renal function; at 70, renal function is, at best, 50% of its original maximum • decreased glomerular filtration rate and tubular secretion lead to an increased possibility of accumulation of all drugs and metabolites eliminated via the kidneys N.B. NSAIDs can accelerate the decline in renal function, particularly in the presence of cardiac failure. Avoid, if possible

Table 24.2 The normal ageing process – changes in nutrition and tissue responses.

Nutrition intake changes	Tissue response changes
• vitamins decrease • proteins decrease • nicotine intake unchanged • alcohol intake unchanged	• reduction of brain cells increases effects of psychoactive drugs • reduction of baroreceptor activity increases postural hypotensive effect of drugs • exaggerated response to anticoagulants; increased risk of gastro-intestinal bleeding with NSAIDs

Table 24.3 The normal ageing process – changes in body composition.

Changes in body composition	Result
• decreased body weight • decreased body water • increased body fat percentage • decreased plasma albumin	• increased effect of standard dose • increased plasma concentration of water-soluble drugs • decreased plasma concentration of fat-soluble drugs • reduced protein binding

Poor nutrition

It is clearly impossible for nurses, pharmacists and family doctors to be aware of the nutritional status of all their elderly patients, but it is essential to run a mental checklist of nutritional changes whenever prescribing for the elderly (*see* Table 24.2).

The community dietitian should be asked to survey the nutritional status of less healthy elderly patients on chronic medication and be asked about and involved in treatment planning and follow-up. Help may be needed at mealtimes.

Changes in tissue responses and body composition

The elderly have increased tissue sensitivity to several commonly needed CNS and cardiovascular drug groups, including the opioid analgesics, the antipsychotics, the anti-Parkinsonian drugs, the benzodiazepines and digoxin (*see* Table 24.2). The *BNF* clearly indicates which drugs require dosage reduction in the elderly, and some drugs have geriatric formulations, for example digoxin 62.5 micrograms.

Body composition changes are also important to remember, particularly in patients aged over 75 years, as the reductions in body weight, body water and plasma albumin all conspire to increase the plasma drug concentration and the effect of many medicines (*see* Table 24.3).

Therefore, it is clear that prescribing for the elderly requires a thorough knowledge of the practical pharmacology that this book has attempted to bring to the prescriber.

Suggestions for rational geriatric prescribing

Box 24.2 lists points to consider when prescribing for senior citizens, particularly if you are considering prescribing a hypnotic, diuretic, NSAID, digoxin, antihypertensive, anti-Parkinsonian, a psychotropic drug or warfarin.

Box 24.3 lists questions for every medication review, which should be conducted at the time of the patient's annual clinical review, or more often if indicated.

Prescribers should be aware of the common problem of co-morbidity in the elderly, leading to unavoidable polypharmacy. This problem is now compounded for the prescriber by the advent of compelling research-based evidence showing the proven benefits of many drug treatments.

This evidence may indicate that a given patient should be prescribed digoxin, a loop diuretic, an ACE inhibitor, a low-dose cardioselective beta-blocker, warfarin *and* a statin, for example. However, the risk of a serious ADR (*see* Chapters 26 and 27) from such an evidence-based combination is greater than 50%, so the decision to prescribe particular treatments and omit others has to be based on experience and knowledge of the patient, as well as research evidence. Such a decision is perhaps best made in consultation with a geriatrician.

Box 24.2 Points to consider when prescribing for elderly patients.

- What is his or her biological age, i.e. is the patient fit for his or her age or should special care with medication be taken due to overt organ failure?
- Should a low starting dose be used (e.g. calcium-channel blockers, many anti-depressants, all benzodiazepines)?
- Has this drug a small margin of safety (e.g. digoxin, theophylline, lithium, warfarin)?
- What is its route of elimination (e.g. avoid chlorpropamide and glibenclamide in any degree of renal impairment)?
- What interactions may occur with the existing treatment?
- Could the new drug worsen existing pathology (e.g. NSAIDs)?

Box 24.3 Questions to consider when reviewing the current long-term drug treatment of elderly patients.

• Is it strictly necessary?	If not, stop.
• Is it being taken?	If not, find out why.
• Are there side-effects?	Discuss with patient.
• Is it having any therapeutic effect?	If not, stop.
• Are any of the drugs incompatible?	If so, stop one.
• Are there signs of drug:drug interaction?	If so, adjust regimen.

Box 24.4 gives suggested general rules for the prescriber when treating elderly patients. Boxes 24.2–24.4, if followed, could improve the health and well-being of your ailing elderly patients, reduce your workload, and greatly reduce the iatrogenic* admission rate mentioned at the beginning of this chapter. You may think them worth copying for your practice team.

---

* iatrogenic = caused by the prescriber

Box 24.4 Some rules for prescribers when treating the elderly.

- Keep prescribing simple – as few drugs as possible, but polypharmacy may be unavoidable (*see* Box 24.1).
- Once- or twice-daily regimens may improve compliance, particularly if associated with mealtimes.
- Encourage a balanced diet – meals on wheels, dietitian, carer.
- Reduce smoking and alcohol intake as much as possible.
- Clear, large labelling is essential.
- Small tablets make swallowing easier.
- Avoid modified-release (SR, LA) products unless they are pharmacologically justified, e.g. the short half-lives of nifedipine and diltiazem make them unsuitable for use except in the SR/LA formulation; note that when prescribing maintenance treatment using any SR/LA formulation, the same brand name should always be used due to variations in pharmacokinetics between brands.
- Avoid fixed-dose combinations, unless they aid compliance.
- Do not use NSAIDs for analgesia only. They are dangerous for the aged.
- Consider the individual's biological age, not chronological age.
- Expect adverse drug reactions and interactions in the elderly – seek them actively.
- Co-operate with the patient, the carer, the nurse, the dietitian and the pharmacist, to foster compliance at every opportunity.

Conclusion

Prescribing for the elderly is probably the most scientifically demanding area of primary care, but the benefits for the patient and the intellectual satisfaction for the prescriber are well worth the effort. 'At the very least, we should do no harm' (Hippocrates of Kos).

The Royal College of Physicians' report on prescribing for the elderly covers this subject in great detail.[5]

Key points

- 27% of all reported adverse drug events occur in the elderly.
- 10–12% of all acute (emergency) hospital admissions in the over-70s are caused by prescribed drugs.
- The anatomical and physiological changes of ageing (listed in this chapter) are partly responsible for these problems.
- The evidence-based co-prescribing of several drugs to treat degenerative disease is another major factor.
- Confusion and poor compliance often contribute.
- The prescriber must select drugs and adjust dosages to take into account reduced liver and kidney function, body composition changes, deficient nutrition and altered tissue responses in the elderly.
- General guidelines are presented in tabular form.

References

1 Pirohamed M, Breckenridge AM, Kitteringham NR *et al.* (1998) Adverse drug reactions. *British Medical Journal.* **316**: 1295–8.
2 Williamson J and Chaplin JM (1980) Adverse drug reactions to prescribed drugs in the elderly: a multicentre investigation. *Age and Ageing.* **9**: 73–80.
3 Ebbeson J, Buajordet I, Erikssen J *et al.* (2001) Drug-related deaths in a department of internal medicine. *Archives of Internal Medicine.* **161**: 2317–23.
4 Huang B, Bachmann KA, Xuming HE *et al.* (2002) Inappropriate prescriptions for the aging population of the United States. *Pharmacoepidemiology and Drug Safety.* **11**: 127–34.
5 Royal College of Physicians (1997) *Medication for Older People* (2e). Royal College of Physicians, London.

25　Antibacterial action and bacterial resistance

In almost all age groups, antibacterials are the most frequently prescribed drugs in general practice.[1] For five decades, we have had the previously unheard-of power to combat almost all bacterial infections. Unfortunately, this 'antibacterial era' is now under serious threat, and will come to an end within the next 5 years if changes are not made.

Already, patients in hospital are dying of systemic infections resistant to all antibacterials. Moreover, common pathogens, such as the *Staphylococci* (many), *Pneumococcus*, *Streptococcus pyogenes*, *Helicobacter pylori*, *Mycobacterium tuberculosis* and *Neisseria gonorrhoeae*, among others, are showing increasing levels of multi-drug resistance in the community.

In this chapter, we shall consider the differences in structure and function of the bacterial cell from that of the human host cell, and how these differences are exploited by antibacterials. Then we will deal with the different types of antibacterial resistance, and how these are transferred within and between bacterial populations.

The scientific use of antibacterials depends on a thorough understanding of these principles.

Bacterial and human cells – vive la différence!
(see Figure 25.1)

Mammalian cells are much more complex than bacterial cells. The evolutionary proliferation of organelles in human cells has resulted in biochemical functions several orders of magnitude more complex than those of bacteria.

Yet bacterial structure and function are highly refined and have adapted the many thousands of bacterial species to life in every known environment: geological, botanical and zoological, including, of course, the human body. Billions of bacteria live in the human body symbiotically, and occasionally as pathogens, causing local and systemic infections.

Antibacterial drugs exploit the differences between bacterial and human cell structure in order to avoid affecting the human host cells, although there are some risks to patients (*see* Figure 25.1 and Table 25.1).

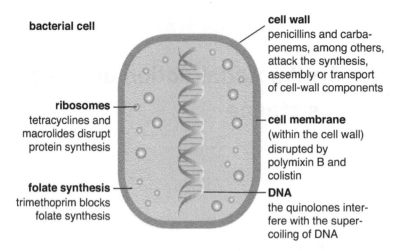

bacterial cell

ribosomes
tetracyclines and
macrolides disrupt
protein synthesis

folate synthesis
trimethoprim blocks
folate synthesis

cell wall
penicillins and carba-
penems, among others,
attack the synthesis,
assembly or transport
of cell-wall components

cell membrane
(within the cell wall)
disrupted by
polymixin B and
colistin

DNA
the quinolones inter-
fere with the super-
coiling of DNA

Figure 25.1 Antibacterial targets in the bacterial cell, and examples of the antibacterials that act at these sites (*see also* Table 25.1).

No bacterial nucleus or organelles

The most obvious difference between human and bacterial cells is that the bacterium has no nucleus, mitochondria, Golgi apparatus or endoplasmic reticulum. Instead, it has a single chromosome without a nuclear membrane, which consists of a tightly wound (supercoiled) DNA molecule lying within the bacterial cytoplasm.

Enzymes control the local uncoiling and recoiling of the chromosome so that biological functions can occur. Some antibacterials, such as ciprofloxacin, block the action of the enzyme topoisomerase II, which is just such a DNA gyrase (*see* Table 25.1).

The rigid bacterial cell wall

Another major target for antibacterials is the cell wall. Although both human and bacterial cells have a phospholipid cell membrane, almost all bacteria have an additional, relatively rigid, outer cell wall. The function of the cell wall is to support the underlying cell membrane, which is under high osmotic pressure and would otherwise burst.

The key component of the cell wall is a substance called peptidoglycan, which is unique to bacteria, and can therefore be exploited by many antibacterials (*see* Table 25.1). These antibacterials disrupt the synthesis or assembly of cell wall components at various sites, or their transport out of the cell.

The cell wall target becomes more complex, however, when Gram-negative bacteria are taken into consideration. These have an additional lipoprotein and lipopolysaccharide membrane outside the cell wall, which is impermeable to a wide variety of antibacterials. By contrast, Gram-positive bacteria do not have an external membrane, and can therefore be more easily affected by the antibacterial mechanisms described above. The bacterial cell membrane can also be attacked directly and disrupted by so-called 'detergent antibacterials', such as the polymyxins.

Table 25.1 How and where antibacterials attack bacteria.

Bacterial structure	Antibacterials that attack this target	Mode of action
bacterial cell wall (peptidoglycan)	penicillins, monobactams, carbapenems, cephalosporins and cephamycin	prevent cross-linkage of peptidoglycan, preventing bacterial cell wall completion
	vancomycin, teicoplanin	inhibit addition of bacterial wall components
bacterial cell membrane	polymyxin B and colistin	disrupt bacterial cell membrane via a 'detergent' action
bacterial protein synthesis (via messenger RNA)	tetracyclines, erythromycin and other macrolides, chloramphenicol, neomycin, streptomycin and other aminoglycosides	disrupt a specific step of bacterial protein synthesis
	rifampicin and other rifamycins	inhibit bacterial RNA polymerase, preventing its transcription to code protein synthesis
bacterial chromosome	ciprofloxacin and other quinolones	disrupt supercoiling of the bacterial chromosome by inhibiting DNA-gyrase
	trimethoprim, sulphonamides	disrupt folate synthesis, thus preventing DNA synthesis

Bacterial protein synthesis

Protein synthesis on messenger RNA templates is different in bacterial and human cells. The tetracyclines, aminoglycosides (e.g. streptomycin), chloramphenicol and the macrolides (e.g. erythromycin), among others, exploit this difference at one or more of the six steps in the protein-assembly process.

The rifamycins (e.g. rifampicin) and metronidazole interfere with aspects of DNA and RNA function, such as metabolism and reproduction.

The bacterial folate synthesis mechanism

Lastly, the commonly used folate antagonist trimethoprim, and the occasionally used sulphonamides, block the synthesis of folate within the bacterium, prior to its use in DNA synthesis. This action effectively blocks DNA function at its earliest stage.

It is clear then that there are several ways in which antibacterials can disrupt bacterial function. Bacteria, however, are able to evolve quickly and can develop resistance to these attacks.

Natural selection – the biological imperative

Bacteria, like all living organisms, undergo occasional mutations, a small proportion of which result in new strains that are more able to resist antibacterial attack. Because of the size of bacterial populations – there are probably more bacteria in the human intestine than there are cells in the human body – and because of their frequency of replication – often once every 20 minutes – the opportunity for developing resistance is enormous. It is unlikely that any antibacterial will be discovered to which bacteria will not develop resistance.

Resistance to antibacterials is promoted by the widespread use of antibacterials, by underdosing and by prolonged courses of treatment. In particular, the unnecessary use of antibacterials for trivial, self-limiting and often viral infections of the upper respiratory tract is a perfect recipe for resistance development. Transfer of resistant bacteria is aided by inadequate hygiene in hospitals, poor infection control techniques, and the close proximity of hospital patients.

The mutant resistant bacteria are often inherently weaker in metabolism than the original 'wild' strains, and cannot establish themselves against the stronger original bacteria. Therefore, resistant bacteria become a very small fraction of the bacterial flora. However, if an antibacterial is prescribed to a patient, the resistant strain has an enormous advantage: the original bacteria will be eliminated and entirely replaced by a population of the resistant strain.

There is also evidence that natural, commensal bacteria have a role in resisting colonisation of the human host by pathogens; for example, commensal *Neisseria* populating the healthy nasopharynx appear to inhibit colonisation by meningococci. This 'colonisation resistance' is an under-recognised defence mechanism. In this and other body areas, e.g. the colon, the use of antibacterials will strip the tissue of its normal, protective flora and facilitate access by pathogens.

How resistance is transferred

Unfortunately, mutations conferring resistance to antibacterials are not restricted to the descendants of the original mutant. The resistance gene can be shared with non-resistant bacteria of the same species and is sometimes transferred to entirely different bacterial strains.

This process is known as 'acquired resistance', and is at the core of the problem of antibacterial resistance. It can occur when:

- there is conjugation between bacteria of the same species and strain, which is when resistant genes (DNA) are passed across interconnecting tubules via plasmids. The gene is not incorporated in the bacterial chromosome (*see* Figure 25.2 ①), but since plasmids self-replicate independently of the bacterial chromosome, resistance genes can be transferred very rapidly by this method

- the resistant gene is incorporated into a neighbouring bacterium's chromosome. In this case, the resistant gene is now permanent and will be transferred to all future generations. This occurs when the resistant gene is transferred across a tubule by a transposon (a section of plasmid DNA), which can insert the resistant gene into the bacterial chromosome. Transposons can carry resistant genes between entirely different bacterial species (*see* Figure 25.2 ②)

- resistance to many antibacterials, known as 'multi-drug resistance', is transferred between bacteria of the same strain and species or to other bacterial species by multi-cassette arrays of genes resistant to many antibacterials. This is a complex, elegant and probably unique biological process, and examples include the notorious methicillin-resistant *Staphylococcus aureus* (MRSA), which is multi-drug resistant and caused over 6000 deaths in the UK in 2008, and the permanent disablement of five times that number (*see* Table 25.2).

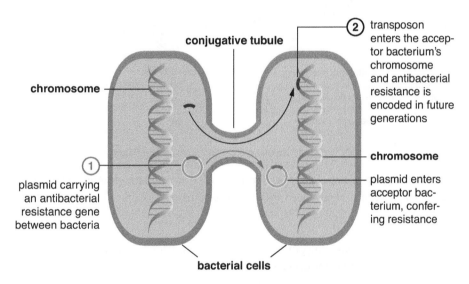

Figure 25.2 Two methods of transfer of antibacterial resistance between bacteria.

The metabolic mechanisms of antibacterial resistance

It remains to describe the biochemical and metabolic processes by which bacteria resist attack by different antibacterials. Once in place, the resistant genes alter the bacterial metabolism in one of five ways, as discussed below (*see* Figure 25.3).[2] Although several hundred different antibacterial resistances have been identified, almost all can be ascribed to one or other of these five classes of resistance.[2]

Enzymatic inactivation (see Figure 25.3 ①)

Bacteria can inactivate the antibacterial before it enters the bacterial cell. For example, staphylococcal resistance to penicillin is usually due to its ability to secrete beta-lactamase, which splits the penicillin molecule.

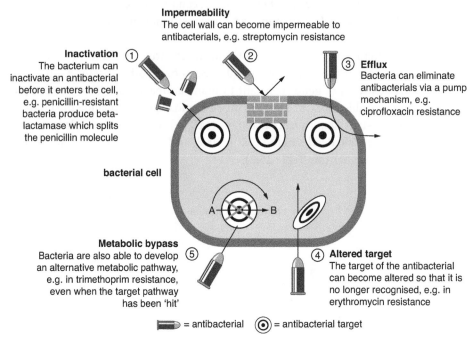

Impermeability
The cell wall can become impermeable to antibacterials, e.g. streptomycin resistance

Inactivation ①
The bacterium can inactivate an antibacterial before it enters the cell, e.g. penicillin-resistant bacteria produce beta-lactamase which splits the penicillin molecule

②

③ **Efflux**
Bacteria can eliminate antibacterials via a pump mechanism, e.g. ciprofloxacin resistance

bacterial cell

Metabolic bypass
Bacteria are also able to develop ⑤ an alternative metabolic pathway, e.g. in trimethoprim resistance, even when the target pathway has been 'hit'

④ **Altered target**
The target of the antibacterial can become altered so that it is no longer recognised, e.g. in erythromycin resistance

= antibacterial = antibacterial target

Figure 25.3 The five classes of bacterial resistance. From *Resistance to Antibacterials and Other Microbial Agents*,[2] reproduced with permission from the Controller of Her Majesty's Stationery Office.

It is of some interest, following our discussion of enzyme induction in Chapter 3, that the beta-lactamase enzyme is induced by the presence of minute amounts of any penicillin or other beta-lactam antibacterial, including the cephalosporins.

Beta-lactamase diffuses from the bacterium, through its cell membrane and cell wall, inactivating the antibacterial molecules in its vicinity.

Cell-wall or membrane impermeability (see Figure 25.3 ②)

The bacterial cell wall and/or plasma membrane can become impermeable to the antibacterial, making it ineffective. Examples of this are resistance to the aminoglycosides, the beta-lactams, chloramphenicol and the tetracyclines.

Pump mechanism (see Figure 25.3 ③)

Bacteria can develop a pump mechanism for extruding the antibacterial molecule (efflux). This is a common mechanism of resistance to ciprofloxacin and the other quinolones, as well as the tetracyclines.

Altered target (see Figure 25.3 ④)

The antibacterial's metabolic 'target', e.g. an enzyme within the bacterium, can become altered so that there is no longer a recognition site for the antibacterial. This is the main mechanism of resistance to erythromycin and the other macrolides.

Bypass mechanism (see Figure 25.3 ⑤)

Finally, bacteria can develop an alternative metabolic pathway or 'bypass' when the antibacterial has reached and disabled its metabolic target. The classic example is bacterial resistance to trimethoprim, in which resistant bacteria have developed an alternative pathway for folic acid synthesis that is insensitive to trimethoprim.

What can be done to preserve the 'antibacterial era'?

Unfortunately, in the majority of cases, resistance against current antibacterials is already encoded in the bacterial chromosome and cannot be overcome by any known measures. As already mentioned, although resistant bacteria are generally biologically weaker than the wild strains, following the prescription of antibacterials they multiply rapidly and occupy the newly available habitat within a few days.

In order to delay antibacterials becoming obsolete (*see* Table 25.2), it is generally recommended that antibacterial use by GPs, vets and farmers should be reduced to an unavoidable minimum, i.e. when there is evidence of significant, systemic bacterial infection. The narrowest spectrum drug should be used, according to the practitioner's knowledge of local bacterial sensitivities.

Table 25.2 Examples of valuable antibacterial therapies now lost or imperilled by the spread of resistance.[2]

Organism	Disease	Agents lost or threatened
Pneumococcus	pneumonia, otitis media, meningitis	penicillin; many others
Meningococcus	meningitis, septicaemia	sulphonamides, penicillin
Haemophilus influenzae	meningitis	ampicillin, chloramphenicol
Staphylococcus aureus	wound infection, sepsis	penicillin, penicillinase-resistant penicillins, others
Salmonella typhi	typhoid fever	most relevant agents
Shigella	bacillary dysentery	most relevant agents
Gonococcus	gonorrhoea	sulphonamides, penicillin, tetracycline (ciprofloxacin)
E. coli (coliforms)	urinary infection, septicaemia	ampicillin, trimethoprim, others
Mycobacterium tuberculosis	tuberculosis	up to four*
multi-drug resistant organisms	many hospital-acquired infections, e.g. MRSA, Clostridium difficile	most antibiotics

Four antitubercular drugs must now be used, sometimes more. Serious interactions are common.

Next, hospitals must return to previous stringent hygienic and nursing standards and reintroduce the time-consuming techniques of strict barrier nursing of both infected and vulnerable (non-infected) patients.

Public education must continue in order to change the expectation that antibacterials will be prescribed for minor, self-limiting infections.

For 50 years, unregulated use of many antibacterials by farmers (in animal feed) has undoubtedly been a major driver of resistance. Repeated warnings have been ignored by the authorities, and the damage has been done and is irreversible.[2]

Finally, if new antibacterials are developed, regulatory agencies, such as the Committee on Safety of Medicines (CSM) in the UK, must take stringent measures to ensure that these precious, new and vulnerable resources are restricted in use to hospital patients only, and even then only on the advice of a medical microbiologist.

It is hoped that this chapter has provided a useful understanding of bacteria and antibacterials, which are subjects of great importance in primary and hospital care. Many millions will die when the antibacterial era ends.

> **Key points**
> - Antibacterial drugs exploit four major differences between human and bacterial cells.
> - A given antibacterial disrupts one of these four elements of bacterial structure and function, killing the bacterium without harming the human cells.
> - Bacteria have evolved five distinct metabolic resistance mechanisms to evade antibacterial attack, via mutation of bacterial DNA.
> - A bacterium can transfer its resistance genes to other bacteria of the same species and to bacteria of many other, unrelated species.
> - Genes encoding resistance to many antibacterials have been transferred to many pathogenic bacterial species and are now causing major problems worldwide in managing life-threatening infections.

References

1 Connolly JP and McGavock H (1999) Antibacterial prescribing for respiratory tract infections in general practice. *Pharmacoepidemiology and Drug Safety.* **8**: 95–104.
2 House of Lords Select Committee on Science and Technology (1998) *Resistance to Antibacterials and Other Antimicrobial Agents.* **HL81-II**: 9. HMSO, London. Still an unsurpassed source of well-researched information.

26 How to prevent adverse drug interactions – ADIs

Adverse effects of prescribed drug therapy are now the fourth leading cause of all deaths in the USA and probably in most developed countries.[1,2] Chapters 26 and 27 describe how we can use pharmacological knowledge to become safer prescribers. Safer prescribing involves reducing the incidence of prescription-related acute hospital admissions and deaths,[3] not to mention the unnecessary symptoms and morbidity caused by adverse drug interactions (ADIs). Whenever two or more drugs are prescribed for a patient, the prescriber should always consider whether one drug is known to interact with the other(s) in an adverse (harmful) manner, for that is a very common occurrence.

ADIs can usefully be divided into six categories. Table 26.1 gives examples of each of these categories:

1 interactions occurring during drug absorption
2 interactions occurring during drug distribution
3 interactions between drugs at their site of action
4 additive and antagonistic effects of two drugs
5 interactions occurring during drug metabolism
6 interactions due to mismatching of two drugs' plasma half-lives.

It may be useful to consult Appendix 1 of the *BNF* when reading this chapter, for a plethora of examples will be found in each category. Unfortunately, they are not type-classified, and they include minor as well as important drug:drug interactions. This is the only section of the *BNF* which is not 'user friendly' to the prescriber.

Table 26.1 The main mechanisms of adverse drug interactions.

Phase of drug activity	Mechanisms leading to ADIs	Well-known examples
1 drug absorption	impairment of absorption, leading to therapeutic failure	antacids reduce the absorption of 14 commonly used drugs/groups – see text
2 drug distribution	one drug may displace a second drug from its protein binding	verapamil displaces digoxin
3 at receptors or other sites of action	competition for receptor binding	beta-blockers diminish the effect of the anti-asthmatic beta$_2$ agonists
4 additive and antagonistic effects of two drugs	additive effects	ACE inhibitors and NSAIDs both reduce aldosterone secretion and in combination may cause dangerous hyperkalaemia
	antagonistic effects	treatment failure
5 metabolism	inhibition or induction of cytochrome P450 enzymes	see text for: 11 important ADIs due to enzyme inhibition and 6 due to enzyme induction
6 mismatching of plasma half-lives when two drugs are used simultaneously	rapid excretion of one drug may expose the patient to the adverse effects of the other	failure to give repeated doses of naloxone when treating comatose heroin addicts

Interactions occurring during drug absorption

Antacids

Patients should usually be warned not to take antacids containing aluminium, magnesium or calcium just before or at the same time as other drugs because they may impair absorption. Antacids may also breach enteric coatings that may have been added to prevent inactivation of a drug by stomach acid. *BNF*, Appendix 1 advises that absorption of the following drugs, among others, is reduced in the presence of antacid:

- ACE inhibitors and angiotensin II antagonists
- many commonly used antibiotics, including azithromycin, ciprofloxacin, most tetracyclines, isoniazid and rifampicin

- the anti-epileptics gabapentin and phenytoin
- the antifungals itraconazole and ketoconazole
- the antihistamine fexofenadine, several antimalarials, the phenothiazine antipsychotics, and sulpiride
- the antiviral zalcitabine
- the bisphosphonates
- digoxin
- oral iron
- the proton pump inhibitor lansoprazole.

These are all true drug:drug interactions occurring before either drug has been absorbed. A similar type of reaction occurs if warfarin or digoxin is taken simultaneously with colestyramine, which prevents their absorption.

Grapefruit, grapefruit juice and bitter (Seville) oranges

Chapter 3 describes the important drug-metabolising enzyme group, the cytochrome P450 mono-oxidase system. This is a major element in the body's capacity to deactivate/detoxify almost all drugs and environmental poisons. One of the most potent of this group, CYP3A4 also occurs in the cells of the small intestine's absorbing surface – the villi. Its function is to deactivate a proportion of all foreign chemicals (toxins) before they can be absorbed, including many drugs.

Unfortunately, grapefruit, grapefruit juice and bitter oranges, in modest quantities, inactivate the intestinal CYP3A4. When that happens, a greater dose than normal of many oral drugs is absorbed into the bloodstream. This can lead to excessive plasma drug concentrations. Table 26.2 is a list of some drugs whose absorption is accelerated if the patient consumes grapefruit. Such patients should be regularly warned about the risk – several of these drugs are highly toxic in overdose.

Finally, drugs that slow gastric emptying will reduce the rate of absorption of most orally administered drugs. The commonest examples of this in practice are the opiate analgesics. Conversely, drugs such as metoclopramide, which speed gastric emptying, will increase the rate of absorption of most drugs.

Table 26.2 Interactions between grapefruit juice and some drugs.

Drug	Possible adverse event	Comments
Amiodarone	Increase in serum amiodarone concentration.	May be clinically significant. Avoid concurrent use.
Atorvastatin	Increased bioavailability of atorvastatin resulting in increased risk of myopathy or rhabdomyolysis.	May be clinically significant.
Carbamazepine	Increased carbamazepine bioavailability.	May be clinically significant. Avoid concurrent use.
Ciclosporin	Increased risk of ciclosporin toxicity (e.g. renal dysfunction, cholestasis, paraesthesia).	Clinically significant interaction. Avoid concurrent use.
Felodipine	Increased serum concentrations may result in increased hypotensive effects or headaches.	May be clinically significant. Avoid concurrent use.
Methylprednisolone	Increased plasma concentrations of methylprednisolone but the extent to which this increases the risk of toxicity is not established.	Monitor if patient drinks large amounts of grapefruit juice.
Midazolam	Increased bioavailability and pharmacodynamic effects of midazolam, e.g. drowsiness.	Avoid concurrent use.
Nicardipine	Increased serum concentrations.	Little change in haemodynamic effect.
Nifedipine	Increased serum concentrations increasing the risk of adverse effects in some patients.	Avoid concurrent use.
Nimodipine	Increased nimodipine plasma concentration.	Avoid concurrent use.
Quinidine	Slight change in quinidine metabolism.	Clinical significance unknown.

(continued)

Drug	Possible adverse event	Comments
Saquinavir	Increased bioavailability.	Clinical significance unknown. Monitor patients for altered response.
Sertraline	May increase serum concentrations.	Clinical significance unclear. Monitor patients for altered response.
Sildenafil **Tadalafil** **Vardenafil**	May increase plasma concentrations.	Avoid concurrent use.
Simvastatin	Increased serum simvastatin concentrations resulting in increased adverse effects (e.g. myopathy, rhabdomyolysis).	May be clinically significant. Avoid concurrent use.
Sirolimus	Increased plasma concentrations resulting in an increased risk of toxicity.	May be clinically significant. Avoid concurrent use.
Tacrolimus	Significantly increased plasma concentrations and increased risk of toxicity.	May be clinically significant. Avoid concurrent use.
Triazolam	Increased serum triazolam concentrations resulting in increased sedation.	Avoid concurrent use.
Warfarin	Possible increased anticoagulant effect.	Limited data.

Interactions occurring during drug distribution

Many drugs are loosely bound to plasma and tissue proteins during distribution to their effector sites. Where two drugs compete for the same protein-binding sites, one may displace the other from its protein binding, releasing it as active free drug in the plasma. This is usually a transient process of no therapeutic significance; however, verapamil or amiodarone cause displacement of digoxin from protein-binding sites leading to digoxin toxicity.

Likewise, giving aspirin or valproate to a patient stabilised on phenytoin increases the free phenytoin concentration, which may cause short-term toxicity, although this is soon corrected by excretion.

Interactions between two drugs at the site of action

Where two drugs compete for binding sites at the same receptor, ion channel, enzyme or carrier mechanism, a reaction may occur.

The classic example is that cardioselective beta-blockers, despite their selectivity for beta$_1$ receptors, which predominate in the heart, still bind to a proportion of beta$_2$ adrenergic receptors in the lungs. This may not only precipitate asthma, but also block the binding of beta agonists, such as salbutamol, used in managing an acute asthmatic attack. Such reactions are avoidable, since they can be predicted from knowledge of the drugs' actions.

Additive and antagonistic effects of two drugs

Drugs with different pharmacological actions but similar therapeutic effects are often used together because of their additive effect. A good example is in the treatment of refractory hypertension, where modern guidelines recommend the use of moderate doses of two or more different antihypertensives rather than a maximum dose of a single drug, e.g. the combination of a calcium-channel blocker and an ACE inhibitor.

Another important example is the treatment of proven rheumatoid arthritis, where the combination of an NSAID with one of several disease-modifying antirheumatic drugs (DMARDs) like azathioprine, ciclosporin or methotrexate is often more effective than an NSAID alone. The additive effect is also used in the drug treatment of many cancers.

However, additive effects can also be dangerous, as in the use of ACE inhibitors and NSAIDs, where both drugs reduce aldosterone secretion and in combination may cause dangerous hyperkalaemia. Moreover, drugs that are mildly sedative on their own may cause significant sedation when combined. By the same token some drugs also cancel another drug's effects, for example NSAIDs reduce the efficacy of all antihypertensives, an example of antagonism.

Drug interactions occurring during drug metabolism

The majority of drugs are metabolised in the liver by the bank of isoenzymes collectively known as the cytochrome P450 oxidases (CYP), which usually render the drug inactive or less active and prepare it for renal excretion (*see* Chapter 3). Unfortunately, a number of important drugs slow down (inhibit) or speed up (induce) one or more of the CYP enzymatic cycles.

Clearly, inhibition of metabolic enzymes will reduce the rate of elimination of the drugs that those enzymes process, and lead to their build-up in the plasma. Enzyme inducers, conversely, will speed up the elimination of the relevant drugs, leading to therapeutic failure. Inhibition and induction of metabolic enzymes are important causes of serious adverse drug reactions and interactions, which may lead to emergency hospital admissions.

Table 26.3 shows 13 major P450 enzyme inhibitors (left column) and some of the commonly used drugs whose metabolism is retarded, leading to increased plasma concentrations, often risky, sometimes life-threatening.

Table 26.4 does the same for the eight major P450 enzyme inducers (left column) and the many drugs whose metabolism is accelerated, leading to lower plasma concentrations and the probability of treatment failure.

These tables are an extension of Tables 3.2 and 3.3 in Chapter 3.

Table 26.3 Metabolic enzyme inhibitors frequently used in primary care: these *increase the effect* of drugs whose metabolism is inhibited. This list is not exclusive.

P450 enzyme inhibitor	Drugs whose plasma concentration is increased
imidazole antifungals, e.g. fluconazole, itraconazole, ketoconazole, etc.	acenocoumarol (nicoumalone), alfentanil, antivirals, ciclosporin, corticosteroids, digoxin, felodipine, midazolam, phenytoin, quinidine, rifabutin, sildenafil, etc., sulfonylureas, tacrolimus, theophylline, warfarin, atypical antipsychotics, valdecoxib, terfenadine, calcium-channel blockers, triptans, cilostazol, new antimalarials
cimetidine	• antihelmintics • anti-arrhythmics: amiodarone, flecainide, lidocaine (lignocaine), procainamide, propafenone, quinidine • antibacterials: erythromycin, metronidazole • anticoagulants: acenocoumarol, warfarin • antidepressants: amitriptyline, doxepin, moclobemide, nortriptyline • anti-epileptics: carbamazepine, phenytoin, valproate • antifungals: terbinafine • antihistamines: loratadine • antimalarials: chloroquine, quinine • anxiolytics and hypnotics: benzodiazepines, clomethiazole • beta-blockers: labetalol, propranolol • calcium-channel blockers: some • cytotoxics: fluorouracil • immunosuppressant: ciclosporin (possibly) • NSAIDs: azapropazone (possibly) • opioid analgesics: pethidine • theophylline
omeprazole	diazepam, digoxin (possibly), clopidogrel
lansoprazole	cilostazol, clarithromycin, phenytoin, methotrexate, tacrolimus
allopurinol	ciclosporin, azathioprine, mercaptopurine, theophylline

(continued)

P450 enzyme inhibitor	Drugs whose plasma concentration is increased
erythromycin and other macrolides	alfentanil, amiodarone, bromocriptine, cabergoline, carbamazepine, ciclosporin, clozapine, disopyramide, felodipine, midazolam, rifabutin, sildenafil, terfenadine, theophylline, zopiclone, moxifloxacin, repaglinide, itraconazole, mizolastine, loratadine, atypical antipsychotics, buspirone, zopiclone, digoxin, some statins
ciprofloxacin, norfloxacin	theophylline, methotrexate
sulphonamides	phenytoin
amiodarone*	acenocoumarol, ciclosporin, digoxin, flecainide, phenytoin, procainamide, warfarin, dabigatran, fidaxomicin
metronidazole	phenytoin, fluorouracil, primidone, lithium or alcohol
SSRIs	benzodiazepines (some), carbamazepine, clozapine, flecainide, haloperidol, phenytoin, propranolol, theophylline, tricyclic antidepressants, ropivacaine, NSAIDs, methadone, many antipsychotics, atomoxetine
calcium-channel blockers – verapamil, diltiazem	alcohol, ciclosporin, digoxin, imipramine, midazolam, nifedipine, phenytoin, quinidine, theophylline, buspirone, cilostazol, dutasteride, sirolimus
several antivirals: indinavir, ritonavir, nelfinavir, saquinavir (see BNF, Appendix 1, under individual drugs for comprehensive list)	erection enhancers (sildenafil, vardenafil, tadalafil), many common analgesics (all NSAIDs, morphine, diamorphine, fentanyl, pethidine, dextropropoxyphene), anti-arrhythmics (amiodarone, flecainide, quinidine, disopyramide, mexiletine, propafenone), macrolide antibiotics (erythromycin, azithromycin, clarithromycin), the SSRI and tricyclic antidepressants, the azole antifungals (itraconazole, ketoconazole), most antipsychotics, most benzodiazepine sedatives, terfenadine, tolterodine, the lipid regulators (atorvastatin, simvastatin)
grapefruit juice and fresh grapefruit (most patients on long-term medication should avoid these, as a precaution)	calcium-channel blockers (nifedipine, felodipine, verapamil, etc.), erection enhancers (as above), anti-rejection immunosuppressants (ciclosporin, sirolimus, tacrolimus), simvastatin, buspirone, terfenadine, efavirenz, saquinavir, atorvastatin, amiodarone, astemizole, carbamazepine, midazolam, sertraline, triazolam, warfarin
ethyl alcohol	enhances the effect of many drugs (not necessary via P450 inhibition). See full page in BNF, Appendix 1 – you will be amazed and enlightened! See below.

* see BNF, Appendix 1, for the many other drug:drug interactions of amiodarone. It is a very 'dirty' drug, but a very effective one. It has a very long half-life – up to 100 days.

It would do no harm to keep Tables 26.3 and 26.4 as an aide-mémoire to be consulted whenever co-prescribing any drug to a patient who is receiving one of the drugs in the left-hand column of either table. But these tables are not comprehensive, and, as always, the *BNF*, Appendix 1 is the definitive source of information on drug interactions. Regular use of primary-care computer software to screen for drug:drug interactions is advisable, and is by far the quickest way to screen for drug:drug compatibility. Your Regional Medicines Information Service is the ultimate source – see front cover of *BNF*.

Table 26.4 Metabolic enzyme inducers: these *reduce the effect* of drugs whose metabolism is accelerated. This list is not comprehensive.

P450 enzyme inducer	Drugs whose plasma concentration is reduced
barbiturates and primidone*	acenocoumarol (nicoumalone), chloramphenicol, ciclosporin, corticosteroids, digitoxin, disopyramide, doxycycline, gestrinone, indinavir, lamotrigine, levothyroxine (thyroxine), metronidazole, mianserin, oral contraceptives, quinidine, theophylline, tibolone, toremifene, tricyclics, warfarin
phenytoin*	acenocoumarol, ciclosporin, clozapine, corticosteroids, digitoxin, disopyramide, indinavir, itraconazole, ketoconazole, lamotrigine, methadone, mexiletine, mianserin, oral contraceptives, paroxetine, quetiapine, quinidine, theophylline, thyroxine, warfarin
carbamazepine*	acenocoumarol, antiepileptics, ciclosporin, corticosteroids, digitoxin, gestrinone, haloperidol, indinavir, mianserin, olanzapine, oral contraceptives, risperidone, theophylline, tibolone, toremifene, tricyclic antidepressants, warfarin
rifamycins	acenocoumarol, amprenavir, atovaquone, benzodiazepines, bisoprolol, carbamazepine, chloramphenicol, chlorpropamide, ciclosporin, cimetidine, corticosteroids, dapsone, digitoxin, diltiazem, disopyramide, fluconazole, fluvastatin, haloperidol, indinavir, itraconazole, ketoconazole, levothyroxine, methadone, mexiletine, nelfinavir, nifedipine, oral contraceptives, phenytoin, propafenone, propranolol, quinidine, simvastatin, sirolimus, tacrolimus, terbinafine, theophylline, tolbutamide, tricyclic antidepressants, verapamil, warfarin
Two antivirals:	
efavirenz	methadone, rifabutin, sertraline, other antivirals (*see BNF*), oestrogens (risking contraceptive failure)
nevirapine	methadone, warfarin, ketoconazole, other antivirals (*see BNF*), oestrogens and progestogens (risk of contraceptive failure)

(*continued*)

P450 enzyme inducer	Drugs whose plasma concentration is reduced
St John's Wort – a very common self-medication herbal. Advise all patients on long-term treatment not to use it	many antivirals, telithromycin, warfarin, amitriptyline, carbamazepine, phenytoin, primidone, phenobarbitone, digoxin, simvastatin, theophylline, tacrolimus, ciclosporin, oestrogens and progestogens (risk of contraceptive failure)
SSRI antidepressants – fluoxetine fluvoxamine sertraline	haloperidol, thioridazine, many atypical antipsychotics, some antivirals
griseofulvin	acenocoumarol, ciclosporin, oral contraceptives, warfarin

*Combination therapy with two or more anti-epileptic drugs enhances toxicity, and drug interactions may occur between anti-epileptics (see BNF, Appendix 1, anti-epileptics).

Interactions due to mismatching of two drugs' plasma half-lives

When two drugs are used together or a drug is used to treat the adverse effects of another drug, it is important to bear in mind the drugs' half-lives. The classic example, not uncommon in present-day emergency care in the community, is the use of naloxone to treat the stuporose or comatose heroin addict. Naloxone displaces morphine and heroin from opioid mu receptors, and very rapidly reverses opioid toxicity, relieving respiratory depression, hypotension, convulsions and sedation, within minutes.

Unfortunately, the half-life of naloxone is only half to one hour, whereas that of heroin is three to four hours. As soon as the naloxone has been metabolised and excreted, the circulating heroin reoccupies the opioid receptors and the dangerous adverse effects recur. That is why it is essential for a prescriber to have several ampoules of naloxone in his or her emergency bag, as it must be repeated according to clinical need.

A further example of mismatching half-lives is the combined use of a thiazide diuretic with amiloride. The two act logically and synergistically in managing mild hypertension, but are strongly associated with the occurrence of fatal hyponatraemia in elderly patients. The reason for this is that amiloride conserves potassium, but increases sodium excretion in the kidneys, with a half-life of 20 hours. This effect is reversed by the thiazide, but the thiazide half-life is only 2.5 hours. Therefore for the remaining 17.5 hours of the daily combined dose, there is a relatively unchallenged sodium loss, which over months can result in profound sodium depletion, collapse, emergency admission, and often death.

If such combinations are used, it is essential to carry out regular plasma electrolyte estimations.

Alcohol (ethanol) – a caution

The majority of Western populations drink alcohol, some people excessively, some moderately and some sparingly. This is important for the prescriber, because alcohol has paradoxical effects on a metabolising cytochrome P450 liver enzyme.

1 Occasional drinking *inhibits* this enzyme (reducing the metabolism of many drugs and leading to an increase in their plasma concentration). The *BNF* (Appendix 1) has two columns citing drugs in this category, whose therapeutic effect is enhanced by concurrent use of alcohol. It includes antihypertensives and antidiabetics. *See BNF* for details.
2 Conversely, chronic, regular drinking *induces* the same enzyme, increasing drug metabolism and leading to reduced plasma concentration and therapeutic failure. The *BNF* fails to describe the reverse effect of alcohol in chronic drinkers and alcoholics. In these patients, there may be a therapeutic failure in the following drugs/groups: warfarin, tolbutamide, doxycycline, antidepressants, antipsychotics, the benzodiazepines and paracetamol.

Beware particularly paracetamol overdosage in chronic drinkers. Because of enzyme induction, their livers produce more of the toxic paracetamol metabolite which often causes death in paracetamol poisoning. Alcoholics should be warned not to take paracetamol.

The disulfiram reaction

The drug disulfiram is sometimes used to help alcoholics to abstain, as it causes most unpleasant symptoms if they drink alcohol – nausea, vomiting, flushing, headache and palpitations. But every prescriber should be aware that a variety of commonly used medicines can also cause this 'disulfiram effect' in some patients if alcohol is taken. These include the cephalosporin antibiotics, the sulphonamides, griseofulvin, nitrofurantoin, metronidazole, isoniazid, the anti-anginal nitrates and the sulfonylurea antidiabetics, tolbutamide, glibenclamide and chlorpropamide.

Patients should be warned accordingly, for the disulfiram reaction can result in cardiovascular collapse, convulsions and death, if the 'dose' of alcohol is very high, as it often is in chronic drinkers.

Conclusion

It is hoped that by using the information from this chapter, prescribers will be aware of the problem and will be able to avoid some ADIs. Information technology is very useful in this area, as it can be used to screen maintenance regimens for interactions, as well as giving the prescriber warnings when he or she is completing a prescription. A good example is the primary care computer software 'EMIS', which will screen a proposed new drug for interaction with a patient's existing medication. Be aware that not all known interactions in the *BNF* are clinically significant. The best software gives some estimate of this. Finally, the pharmacist should always be involved in reviewing long-term medication, dosage adjustment and compliance.[1] Your Regional Medicines Information Service is only a phone-call away – see inside front cover of the *BNF*. Their information will be rapid, updated and will indemnify the prescriber legally, should that be necessary.

The next chapter is concerned with avoiding and dealing with adverse drug reactions due to individual drugs as monotherapy (no other drug treatment).

For further study, *see* reference 4.

Key points

■ Adverse drug interactions (ADIs) occur when one drug affects the absorption, distribution, action or metabolism of a second drug in a manner harmful to the patient.

■ There are six distinct pharmacological categories of ADI.

■ The mechanisms of these are described and examples given.

■ The most serious ADIs are due to induction or inhibition of metabolic enzymes by one drug, causing inadequate or excessive plasma concentrations, respectively, of a second drug.

■ A practice aide-mémoire is provided.

References

1 Hepler CD and Segal R (2003) *Preventing Medication Errors and Improving Drug Therapy Outcomes.* CRC Press, Boca Raton, pp 1–27.

2 Huang B, Bachmann KA, Xuming HE *et al.* (2002) Inappropriate prescriptions for the aging population of the United States: an analysis of the National Ambulatory Medical Care Survey, 1997. *Pharmacoepidemiology and Drug Safety.* **11**: 127–34.

3 McGavock H (2004) Prescription-related illness – a scandalous pandemic. *Journal of Evaluation in Clinical Practice.* **10**(4): 491–7.

4 McGavock H (2009) *Pitfalls in Prescribing and How to Avoid Them.* Radcliffe Publishing, London and New York.

27 How to predict and avoid adverse drug reactions to single drugs – ADRs

In the previous chapter, the different types of adverse drug interaction (ADI) were explored with special reference to their avoidance by GP prescribers. In this chapter, the subject is adverse drug reactions (ADRs) to individual drugs, used as monotherapy (i.e. alone).

Prescribers should be aware that several international classifications of ADRs have been produced for the purposes of epidemiological research and/or drug licensing regulations. These are by no means prescriber friendly, and this chapter aims to help and inform the reader wishing to reduce the risks of ADRs in his or her patients. The topic will be covered in three sections:

1 common, predictable ADRs, i.e. ADRs due to the pharmacological or physiological actions of a drug
2 rare, unpredictable ADRs, i.e. unavoidable, idiosyncratic ADRs with no obvious link to pharmacology or physiology
3 ADRs due to inappropriate prescribing.

Common, predictable ADRs

When any drug is prescribed, there is a possibility of one or more predictable ADRs occurring. As explained in previous chapters, drugs that block or stimulate receptors, ion channels, cellular enzymes or cell-membrane carrier molecules will bind to and affect the function not only of the diseased (target) system, but of every binding site in the body for that drug molecule (*see* Table 27.1).

The result of this unwanted stimulation or blockade at 'non-target' sites is an ADR disrupting the normal physiological regulation of one or many body processes. (Even so-called 'selective' drugs produce such disruption, but usually to a lesser extent than non-selective drugs.) Well-known examples are the tricyclic antidepressants, the SSRIs, and levodopa.

The individual patient's experience of such side-effects and tolerance of them varies greatly, as do patients' reactions to different members of the same therapeutic drug class.

Table 27.1 Some predictable ADRs and their pharmacological basis.

Drug(s)	ADR	Pharmacological cause
antibiotics	diarrhoea, *Clostridium difficile*, colitis, thrush	disruption of normal intestinal flora
beta-blockers	asthma cold extremities heart failure (in standard doses) fatigue (TATT – tired all the time)	bronchoconstriction peripheral vasoconstriction negative inotropic action (reduction of cardiac contractility)
calcium-channel blockers	headache, peripheral oedema, flushing, palpitations, heart block (the latter, diltiazem and verapamil only)	peripheral vasodilatation, blocking of cardiac conducting system
digoxin	cardiac arrhythmias, heart block	slowing of atrio-ventricular (AV) conduction in heart
immunosuppressants	susceptibility to infection, increased risk of cancers	depression of immune system
levodopa	hypomania, psychosis, nausea, vomiting	action on many cerebral dopaminergic neurons
thiazide diuretics	insidious onset of hypokalaemia	small daily excess potassium loss over months
loop diuretics	hypokalaemia, hyponatraemia, hypomagnesaemia, increased calcium excretion, hypotension	diuretic activity (on renal tubules), with 'unbalancing' of ion excretion
NSAIDs	peptic ulcer, acute renal failure, exacerbation of asthma, etc.	blockade of physiological prostaglandin synthesis
tricyclic antidepressants	drowsiness, dry mouth, blurred vision, constipation, urinary retention, cardiac arrhythmias	disruption of autonomic control (antimuscarinic anticholinergic effect)
warfarin	loss of INR* control with bleeding	antagonism of vitamin K enhanced, often due to drug:drug interaction – *see BNF*, Appendix 1

*INR = international normalised ratio, a reliable measure of anticoagulation.

That is why some patients tolerate a particular NSAID, SSRI or oral contraceptive better, and why it is worth trying different analogues to find the preparation that suits an individual best for long-term treatment. However, it is important to remember that these ADRs are predictable and dose related. Table 27.1 gives some well-known examples.

Prostaglandins

A good example of the problems associated with 'blanket' blocking of physiological regulators is the adverse effects due to inhibition of prostanoid production by NSAIDs. Prostanoids have a variety of physiological actions, including mediation of inflammatory response, renal regulation, vasodilatation, inhibition of gastric acid secretion, increased gastric mucus secretion, bronchodilatation and pregnancy (*see* Chapter 8).

By blocking prostanoid production, NSAIDs can have a range of adverse effects, including peptic ulceration, renal failure, and exacerbation of asthma, in addition to their beneficial effects on inflammation.

Serotonin (5-HT)

The same problem arises with drugs that affect important neurotransmitters. Serotonin, like the prostaglandins, has widespread physiological regulatory functions in the gastrointestinal tract, the smooth muscle of the uterus and bronchial tree, the large and small blood vessels (with paradoxical effects), the platelets, the peripheral nerve endings and, of course, the central nervous system (CNS).

Study of the *BNF* monograph on selective serotonin reuptake inhibitors (SSRIs) indicates that ADRs include nausea, dyspepsia, abdominal pain, diarrhoea, constipation, nervousness, anxiety, headache, insomnia, convulsions, sweating, hypomania, etc.[1] Here again, there is great individual variation in susceptibility to and tolerance of any of these ADRs.

Where a patient experiences an unacceptable ADR, reduction of dosage will often bring relief, but may also reduce the plasma concentration of the drug to subtherapeutic levels. In such a case, it is always worth trying a different chemical compound in the same pharmacological class.

Advance warning

All prescribers should be aware of the value of discreetly warning patients in advance that they may experience some side-effects, inviting them to report such side-effects promptly, and having a discussion about them. In many cases, such as the well-known adverse effects of HRT – nausea, breast tenderness, weight gain, fluid retention and headaches – perseverance with the treatment for a few weeks or months will see the physiological readjustment of the body to the drug (often with up- or down-regulation of receptors) and a gradual disappearance of the ADR. HRT = hormone replacement therapy for severe post-menopausal symptoms.

Patients also need to be informed that all drugs have adverse reactions and risks and that there is a trade-off between high probability of benefit and low probability of risk with every prescription, including vaccination. Failure to do so will leave the prescriber legally vulnerable. It remains the clinician's duty to be aware of all the main ADRs and ADIs, and to seek them actively, using symptoms, signs and the monitoring of plasma drug concentrations and other laboratory testing, when necessary – *BNF* specifies when the latter is necessary.

Cessation of treatment

Finally, all prescribers should be aware of the occurrence of adverse reactions on cessation of treatment. This is usually due to the body's compensatory up- or down-regulation of receptors in response to the drug treatment, leading to a 'rebound phenomenon' when treatment ends.

It is common practice to withdraw many drugs gradually, e.g. antipsychotics, antidepressants, opiate analgesia and some antihypertensives. Poorly compliant patients are particularly prone to this type of ADR. The *BNF* gives clear advice on the withdrawal of these medicines, and the pharmacist must label them accordingly.

Rare, unpredictable ADRs – reporting on suspicion

Rare, unpredictable ADRs are sometimes known as 'idiosyncratic, Type B reactions'. They are fortunately rare (often as infrequent as 1 per 100 000 treatment-years) and they cannot be predicted from a drug's known pharmacology.

This means that the postmarketing surveillance of each new medicine depends on the vigilance and spontaneous reporting by doctors, nurses and pharmacists of suspected ADRs via the Department of Health Yellow Card system and the Prescription Event Monitoring scheme run by the Drug Safety Research Unit, Southampton. Type B reactions are often devastating and irreversible and have led to the abandonment of many otherwise useful drugs like thalidomide, practolol, cerivastatin, troglitazone and grepafloxacin. Tear-out yellow cards can be found at the back of every *BNF*. Use them on suspicion – do not await certainty of causality. It is estimated that only one in six serious ADRs is reported spontaneously (the Yellow Card approach).

Pre-existing susceptibility

In all of these cases, there is evidence that a tiny proportion of patients have a genetic, metabolic or physiological susceptibility to the ADR. This certainly applies to the anaphylactic shock caused by penicillin, streptomycin and vaccines in a small proportion of susceptible patients. It also applies to the occurrence of agranulocytosis due to clozapine, carbimazole and chloramphenicol, and the Stevens–Johnson syndrome (major erythema multiforme) due to NSAIDs, phenytoin and sulphonamides.

The need for a high index of suspicion

Some rare ADRs are immunological in origin, i.e. anaphylactic. Their rarity is worth emphasising: you might encounter one of these reactions twice in your career. However, on a national basis, such reactions account for the death of several hundred patients annually in the UK.

The only known response to this risk is the high index of suspicion that characterises the experienced prescriber, instant checking with your regional medicines information service as to the possibility of a causal relationship between the drug and the suspected ADR, and immediate withdrawal of the drug. The sooner such a drug is withdrawn, the more likely the patient's survival.

Unpredictable reactions are not dose-related, and may recur after even a minute dosage. Patients should carry a MedicAlert warning if they have experienced such a reaction in the past, e.g. a survivor of Stevens–Johnson syndrome should carry a warning to avoid the causal agent.

Avoiding ADRs: inappropriate prescribing

A large proportion of ADRs are entirely avoidable. Safe and effective prescribing is dependent on accurate diagnosis, and in primary care this is not always possible. Indeed one of the many skills of the general practitioner is the ability to manage diagnostic uncertainty, based on an assessment of improbability as much as one of probability.

In such circumstances, drugs are sometimes used inappropriately, the commonest example being the prescription of antibiotics for self-limiting infections of the upper respiratory tract in both sexes and all ages. Where the infection is due to a virus (70% of all upper and lower respiratory infections), the patient is exposed to 100% risk with 0% benefit. Other examples are proton pump inhibitors prescribed when only lifestyle changes are needed, NSAIDs given when there is no evidence of any inflammation, and SSRI antidepressants prescribed for mild, short-term depression. These can only be described as bad practice.

Contraindications

Classic examples of inappropriate prescribing are the use of drugs in patients whose diagnosis contraindicates their use. Research in both the USA and the UK has shown that inappropriate drug use may account for as much as 2.5% of all prescribing. A common example is the use of drugs known to precipitate asthma in a patient with a past history of bronchial asthma. Another frequent example is the prescription of any benzodiazepine to a patient with a diagnosis of depression, since all benzodiazepines worsen depressive symptoms.

NSAIDs will cause deterioration in patients with either heart or renal failure. Heart failure and cardiac conduction problems will be exacerbated by prescribing either of the calcium-channel blockers verapamil or diltiazem. For the past 17 years in the USA, the Medicaid service has screened every GP's prescribing monthly, seeking the many examples of inappropriate prescribing, notifying the doctors involved, and preventing potential future harm to patients.

Conclusion

Chapters 26 and 27 have shown that a proportion of ADIs and ADRs are avoidable using the information that this book has tried to convey. It is unlikely that ADRs will ever be completely eliminated, despite the best efforts of the pharmaceutical industry to produce ever more selective and tolerable drugs and the best efforts of clinicians to make their prescribing an applied science, as it is at its best.

Nevertheless, there is no reason why the incidence of serious, life-threatening ADRs and ADIs should not be greatly reduced using pharmacological knowledge. This can be aided by the regular use of information technology to screen for drug interactions, and by involving community pharmacists more directly in long-term patient care, with therapeutic reviews of medication, searches for side-effects and fostering compliance. As previously stated, every prescriber should cultivate a high index of suspicion that a change of symptoms or signs might be due to some aspect of the patient's medication. Bear in mind also that around 40% of patients do not comply with their treatment schedule. That is the commonest cause of treatment failure, but it is also the reason behind about 33% of all prescription-related hospital admissions. The prescriber, the pharmacist, the carer and the patient have a duty to reinforce the compliance message at every opportunity.

The regional or district Medicines Information Service is an excellent source of help when the prescriber is in doubt regarding any medication; the telephone numbers are listed on the inside front cover of the *BNF*. This is a 24-hour service.

In summary, use your pharmacological knowledge to avoid ADRs at the moment of writing the prescription or repeat prescription. Then be proactive in seeking out ADRs in your patients, especially the elderly. Respond quickly and appropriately whenever you suspect them. There is no more important or rewarding area of clinical practice.

Key points

■ ADRs can be divided into two categories: predictable and unpredictable.

■ Predictable ADRs are usually dose-related and due to the known pharmacology of the drug.

■ Some drugs, such as tricyclic antidepressants, cause side-effects due to their action on receptors in organs other than the target.

■ Patients should be warned in advance of well-known adverse reactions, e.g. from HRT, and urged to persevere.

■ Cessation of treatment can bring about adverse reactions, hence the necessity to withdraw some drugs gradually, e.g. opiates, antipsychotics, antidepressants.

■ Unpredictable ADRs are very rare, and can be assigned in some cases to a pre-existing susceptibility in the patient.

■ Drugs such as antibiotics are commonly prescribed inappropriately for self-limiting infections, subjecting patients to risk without benefit.

■ ADRs can occur when drugs are prescribed to patients in whom they are contraindicated (the wrong drug for the stated diagnosis).

■ Screening technology, co-operation of the community pharmacist and vigilance can all help to avoid ADRs.

■ Compliance with drug treatment should be promoted at every opportunity.

Reference

1 BNF, Section 4.3.3. Introductory monograph: Selective serotonin re-uptake inhibitors. BMA/ RPSGB, London.

Further reading

• Rang HP, Dale MM, Ritter JM and Flower RJ (2012) *Pharmacology* (7e). Churchill Livingstone, Oxford. (If you wish to delve more deeply.)
• *British National Formulary* (*BNF*), published yearly. BMA/RPSGB, London. (For regular use.)
• Hardman JG and Limbird L (2001) *Goodman and Gilman's The Pharmacological Basis of Therapeutics* (10e). McGraw-Hill Education, New York. (For occasional reference.)
• McGavock H (2009) *Pitfalls in Prescribing and How to Avoid Them*. Radcliffe Publishing, London and New York.

28 Why consider a practice formulary?

Why?

Chapters 26 and 27 have shown the complexity of modern prescribing. Every year, a dozen or more new drugs become available, all with side-effects, contraindications and

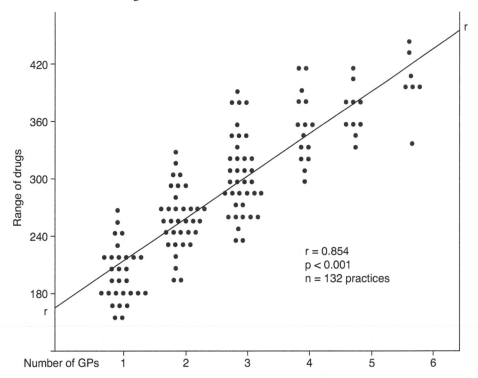

Figure 28.1 Scatterplot showing the relationship between the number of different drugs prescribed by a practice and the number of GPs in that practice. Each dot represents one practice's monthly total. All practices in one small UK region are included. r–r is the regression line.

as yet unknown ADRs and ADIs. Even using information technology to aid prescribing, the intellectual load is too great for even the finest brains.

Research has shown that the average GP uses between 120 and 260 different drugs (average 200), rarely departing from what is, in essence, his or her personal formulary. They 'know' their drugs, caveats, problems and therapeutic results. When we consider partnerships, the number of different drugs rises with each partner, reaching an average of 400 in a group practice of six partners – there is little or no consensus. That cannot be safe, since a patient may be seen by three or four different doctors on successive visits – refer to Chapters 26 and 27.

Please study Figure 28.1 – it shows the rigorous statistical analysis of all GPs in an entire UK region of 132 practices (362 GPs). (Note the high correlation coefficient, r, and significance, p.)

This figure[1] and the previous chapters are surely strong reasons for an agreed practice formulary to be used by all, including locums. Allowance must be made for occasional, justifiable departures from the agreed list (e.g. consultant recommendations). Hundreds of the most quality-minded group practices already have a 'tight' practice formulary. Perhaps all group practices should devise one in the interest of safety and science.

How?

Is making a practice formulary difficult? No, but it requires commitment, effort, negotiation and give-and-take. Here's how . . .

1 Select the nine categories of drug most relevant to general practice – gastro-intestinal, cardiovascular, respiratory, central nervous system, infections, endocrine (including obstetrics and gynaecology), musculo-skeletal, ear, nose and throat and dermatology.
2 Allocate one or more of these categories to each partner, who then becomes the practice 'expert' in those groups.
3 Allow two or three weeks for all partners to draw up a provisional short-list, including a preferred drug selection for each disease, e.g. hypertension, asthma, GORD, depression, joint pains – the *BNF*'s short introduction under each heading is a good starting-point, but reference to an international-quality, up-to-date text will give much more comparative guidance, e.g. *Current Medical Diagnosis and Treatment* (McPhee SJ, Papadakis MA (eds), Lange), published yearly.
4 In the course of this exercise, partners will develop a superior level of knowledge in his or her section(s) and should become the 'partner of reference' for the other partners from then on.
5 Meet weekly for a two-hour discussion – one formulary section per meeting. An independent expert should be present to inform and adjudicate, e.g. a pharmaceutical adviser, a therapeutics and pharmacology lecturer, or a hospital registrar in that specialty. A partner from another practice which runs a formulary could also help.

Such is professional goodwill that it is not usually difficult to recruit such people for a single session.

6 When the sections are all completed and agreed, have the formulary typed up and proofread (time-consuming, but dosages must be correct), then photocopied and bound.

7 Schedule a meeting every six months to (a) discuss problems and (b) amend the formulary, being careful to remove an existing entry if a new drug is to be adopted. Try never to add a newly marketed drug – about one new drug in five is withdrawn due to patient harm, in its first 3–4 years of use.

8 Use your monthly prescribing data for the practice and for each member (and practice nurses) to check for GP adherence and seek reasons for non-adherence, e.g. specialist recommendations.

Within a year, you will wonder how you ever managed without a formulary and should be enjoying prescribing as the rewarding applied science which it is.

Reference

1 McCarthy M, Wilson-Davis K and McGavock H (1992) Relationship between the number of partners in a general practice and the number of different drugs prescribed by that practice. *British Journal of General Practice*. **42**: 10–12.

29 Getting new drugs to market: licensing medicines for human use

If pharmacology is important for the prescriber, it is even more important during the production, testing and licensing of a new drug. Almost the full range of pharmacological knowledge comes into play during this complex process, which can take up to 12 years and cost over £1 billion. The pharmaceutical manufacturer is responsible for all of this preliminary scientific work, at the end of which the company submits a dossier, often running to hundreds of pages in length, to the national drug licensing organisation, e.g. the Medicines and Healthcare Products Regulatory Agency in the UK and the Food and Drugs Administration in the USA.* A typical application comprises the following sections:

1 description of the active chemical compound
2 description of the quality control processes during its manufacture
3 description of the pharmaceutics – the vehicle (e.g. a powder) in which the active substance is carried, the process of tabletting or preparation of capsules or injectate, etc. Excipients may include additives necessary to stabilise the active chemical compound and, in the case of some injections, antiseptic agents to inhibit the growth of micro-organisms
4 description of the mandatory preclinical tests conducted in animal models, including toxicity and carcinogenesis testing
5 description of the clinical trials carried out in human volunteers and patients, of which there are three phases prior to the licensing and marketing of a new drug.

Preclinical testing

The preclinical phase of drug development involves the testing of the new drug in animal models. This is first to determine its action on the likely human target organ and its additional effects on other organs (the pharmacodynamics). Second, there are extensive tests

---

* Every developed country has its own version of the MHPRA and FDA, and there is now a pan-European Community agency.

for toxicity on all the major organ systems, again carried out on suitable animal models. Third, there is the very important and rigorous testing for teratogenicity – the potential to produce cancers. Only after a new drug has cleared all of the research and preclinical hurdles can it be considered for testing in human subjects (*see* Box 29.1).

Box 29.1 The development of new drugs.

Research
Discovery of a new active chemical compound
↓
Preclinical testing
In vitro and animal studies, defining pharmacology and toxicology
↓
Clinical trials (human studies), 4 phases
↓
Phase 1
Volunteer studies (up to 100 healthy people)
Investigating safety, pharmacokinetics and metabolic effects
↓
Phase 2
Controlled studies in a homogeneous group of patients
(up to 500 patients)
Proving safety, efficacy and dosage range
↓
Phase 3
Testing safety and efficacy in a more heterogeneous population
Pivotal clinical trials (up to 3000 patients)
↓
Submission of dossier to licensing authority
↓
Phase 4
Post-marketing surveillance, including:

- ongoing investigation of safety and adverse effects
- establishing efficacy in the general population
- determining cost-effectiveness
- seeking unexpected therapeutic benefits (leading to extension of licence)

Clinical trials: testing a new drug on healthy and sick people

Box 29.1 shows that the clinical trials of a drug are usually grouped in four phases. This is the most critical and commercially risky part of new drug development. The potential of a promising new therapeutic substance to cause harm is a major risk, both to healthy volunteers and to patients with the target disease. As described in previous chapters, drugs are rarely entirely selective for their target receptor, ion channel, enzyme or carrier mechanism, and will affect all similar binding sites, often causing unacceptable side-effects. In addition, there is always the possibility of idiosyncratic adverse reactions, as described in Chapter 27. So volunteers taking part in phases 1, 2 or 3 of clinical trials should be monitored with the utmost care and in the greatest possible detail. All research in phases 1–3 must have independent ethical approval before it can proceed.

Phase 1

In phase 1 of the clinical trials, up to 100 healthy volunteers are given the new drug and subjected to physiological, pharmacological and biochemical tests aimed to reveal safety, side-effects, metabolic effects and, particularly, the pharmacokinetics of the drug as described in Chapters 1–4 of this book. Such volunteer subjects are carefully screened for pre-test normality. In particular, anyone taking any other drug or consuming large amounts of alcohol is excluded, as are any volunteers with any form of detectable biochemical or endocrine abnormality. Subjects are normally paid for their time and in recognition of the risk involved. This phase 1 testing is often done in university departments of pharmacology, or by specialised companies who undertake this work for the product owner.

Phase 2

In phase 2 trials, the new drug is used for the first time in patients suffering from the condition which the drug is expected to benefit, either by rebalancing the disturbed physiology, or by killing cancerous cells or invading micro-organisms. Phase 2 trials are carried out on relatively small numbers – a maximum of 500 patients in most cases – and are usually in the form of randomised, double-blind, controlled clinical trials, in which half of the group receive the new drug while the other half continue to receive their existing treatment or a placebo. Such studies are designed to prove efficacy, to look at safety once again, and to determine the dosage range most likely to be required. Phase 2 studies are unlikely to be predictive of the drug's effects in the general population, because of the exclusions imposed by the overriding need for avoidance of harm. Phase 2 studies, and pre-licensing drug trials generally, exclude the old, children, pregnant women, people taking other drugs, heavy drinkers and smokers, and all drug abusers. So these trials are not conducted on typical primary care patients!

Phase 3

In phase 3 trials, up to 3000 patients with an appropriate diagnosis receive the new drug, usually in the setting of a randomised, blinded, controlled trial lasting anything from three months to a year. From the licensing point of view, phase 3 trials are the most critical, since they are carried out on a relatively heterogeneous population, though with the same exclusions referred to above, and usually in the relatively controllable environment of hospital medicine.

Application to the licensing authority

Following phase 3 clinical trials of a new drug, the parent pharmaceutical company submits a detailed and very lengthy dossier, reporting all the known facts about the new drug in its possession, to the licensing authority. The various sections of this lengthy file are scrutinised by authority experts in each of the relevant fields: pharmaceutical, toxicological, preclinical and clinical, including a rigorous assessment of the statistical procedures that the company has followed in its trials. The licensing authority may grant authorisation, require the company to conduct further proving tests and resubmit its application, or reject the application. In Europe, this process can now be undertaken in a number of ways. First, on a national basis, which involves licensing the drug for a particular country. Second, the company may opt for a centralised procedure, licensing the drug for the entire European Union. Alternatively, a mutual recognition procedure may be followed, in which authorisation by one member state is followed by submission to the other member states, who may or may not approve the new compound.

Phase 4: post-marketing surveillance

Post-marketing surveillance is in every respect as important as phases 1, 2 and 3, and is often a great deal more difficult to conduct. Once a drug is marketed and widely prescribed by clinicians, who may not always have an adequate understanding of its properties (relying on the advice of consultant colleagues or, indeed, of drug industry representatives, for their information) the potential for harm begins to emerge. Added to this is the fact that primary care clinicians are not always as aware of the need for clinical suspicion of adverse events as they might be. It is in phase 4 that the types and incidence of adverse drug reaction and adverse drug interaction are usually defined, a process which may take millions of prescriptions and several years and which may lead to the withdrawal of the drug within a few years of its licensing. On the other hand, post-marketing surveillance may reveal unexpected benefits from a new drug, giving that drug company a marketing advantage. Box 29.1 summarises this long and costly process. Clinical opinion tends to pass through an initial phase of optimism regarding newly licensed drugs – the wonder-drug scenario! If serious adverse effects are revealed, this is often followed by an equally uncritical period of professional distrust, sometimes quite unjustified, as the adverse effects are often related to incorrect use of the new drug. Unfortunately, such distrust may reach a national level, and occasionally result in the withdrawal of a promising new treatment, which if selectively and scientifically used, should have remained available, at least on a consultant-advised basis.

Box 29.2 The golden age of drug innovation, 1960–2015.

- Penicillin esters
- Loop diuretics
- Antipsychotics
- Tricyclic antidepressants
- Benzodiazepines
- Cephalosporins
- 4-Quinolones
- Macrolides
- Oral contraceptives
- Hormone replacement therapy
- Beta-blockers
- NSAIDs
- Beta$_2$-adrenoceptor agonists
- Inhaled steroids
- Histamine H$_2$ receptor blockers
- Anti-emetics
- Synthetic prostaglandin analogues

- Calcium-channel blockers
- ACE inhibitors
- Selective serotonin reuptake inhibitors
- Cancer chemotherapy – many powerful agents now available
- Lipid-lowering agents
- Proton pump inhibitors
- Anti-oestrogens and hypothalamic and pituitary hormones
- New hypoglycaemics
- Anti-androgens
- Monoclonal antibodies
- Antiviral agents
- Selective oestrogen receptor modulators
- Cytokine modulators

The final phase in a new drug's development is the acceptance phase, in which its known benefits are balanced against its known risks, and its position in the therapeutic armamentarium is accepted worldwide.

There are perhaps two lessons for the prescriber resulting from the above account. First, to respect the enterprise and effort of the drug industry which has, over the past 55 years, given us a golden age of drug discovery (*see* Box 29.2). Second, to remember that a new drug should rarely be prescribed in the community without the recommendation of a consultant, and that when it is prescribed, the prescriber is responsible for maintaining a high index of suspicion, and reporting on suspicion alone, any perceived adverse effects to the National Pharmacovigilance Authority, using the 'Yellow Card' at the back of the *BNF*, in the UK.

30 The problem of patients' non-compliance with their medication – 'non-concordance'

Twenty years of drug use research across the 'developed' world have shown consistent and worrying evidence of the extent of the non-compliance (or non-adherence) of patients with their prescribed medication – both short-term courses and long-term regimens. In summary, about 20% of patients take their medications (and medicate their children and older dependents) with remarkable precision, gaining maximal benefit as a result. A further 40% take their medicines with varying degrees of imperfection, but well enough to derive therapeutic benefit, although less than if they had self-medicated more precisely. The remaining 40% do not take their prescribed medicines at all, or they take them so badly that they get no benefit whatsoever – of these, 15% do not even get their prescriptions dispensed!

The psychological and sociological characteristics of these three groups have been thoroughly studied, and they make interesting background reading for the family doctor, aiding a sympathetic understanding of this vagary of human behaviour.[1]

Of more direct relevance to the general practitioner and nurse prescriber is the realisation that these statistics probably apply to *your* practice, and that 40% of *your* patients gain no benefit from your knowledge, skill, care and effort. The ultimate evidence of the effects of non-compliance is the observation that over 90% of organ transplant rejection (and death) is due to non-compliance with the immunosuppressant regimen. And it has often been reported that up to 70% of asthmatic children admitted to A&E with acute, severe asthma have not been receiving their preventive steroid inhalations regularly. Since the near-abandonment of antipsychotic depot injections, the majority of psychotic patients in the community stop their oral medication, then swing into an acute psychotic episode, with all of its personal and societal sequelae, and then restart the drug, forgetting that with every relapse the illness deteriorates further and the prognosis worsens.

Non-compliance involves waste. Apart from the waste of the doctors' and pharmacists' time and expertise, and of the NHS budget (on average, about £25 per prescription item), the failure of non-compliant patients to avail themselves of the benefits of modern pharmacology has serious adverse outcomes. Patients with long-term diseases such as diabetes, hypertension, hyperlipidaemia, asthma, rheumatoid arthritis and schizophrenia, who do not take their medicines properly, deteriorate much earlier in life than they need otherwise do, and die earlier – a waste of life itself and of quality of life. Their hospital re-admission rate is much higher than it should be – a vast waste of NHS beds and resources. It is impossible to be precise, but it is estimated that at least £10 billion is wasted each year in the UK, by non-compliance.

It is important for clinicians to know that a subgroup of the 40% of non-compliers are those who take their maintenance regimens intermittently, with gaps of days or weeks, or who 'cherry-pick' their 'favourite' medicines from a regimen of five or more drugs. They do not realise that their prescription was selected to have a balanced, synergistic, long-term effect. This subgroup is at particular risk due to the phenomenon of up-regulation or down-regulation of cell receptors (*see* Chapter 7), causing over- or under-physiological compensation when a drug is suddenly stopped. Good examples are antihypertensives, SSRI antidepressants and the antipsychotics. The *BNF* clearly advises gradual withdrawal of the latter two drug groups.

For those who wish to know a little more about compliance research findings, there is a short summary at the end of this chapter.

The practical question is 'Can anything be done about non-compliance?'

The answer is that much can be done for the majority of the 40% of non-compliers. Many strategies and tactics have been devised, particularly in the USA.[2] Almost all of them have been proved to work for most patients and to improve outcomes, but only for as long as the intervention has continued. When the intervention is stopped, the patients often revert to their previous behaviour.

That being so, here are some of the most effective compliance-enhancing techniques: many of them involve an extra workload for the prescribing doctor, the nurse, the pharmacist or the carer, or several of them. However, if we are committed to excellence and know that we can substantially improve the care that we give, many of us will be prepared for this extra, paternalistic role of protecting our patients from themselves! If you make that choice, here are some proven and practicable compliance-enhancing methods:

1 *Recognise the problem – diagnose non-compliance.*
If there is no clinical response, reconsider your diagnosis. If the diagnosis is firm, do not increase the dosage immediately. Ask the patient whether they have any problem in taking the medicines, and to tell you how and how often each drug is to be taken. Then remember that many patients have been shown to lie about their compliance (often to avoid offending you), and check with their pharmacist that their prescriptions have been dispensed and collected. Finally, check whether repeat prescriptions are being requested at approximately the expected intervals. This will also reveal 'over-compliance'.

When you are reasonably sure that the patient is non-compliant, it is obviously counter-productive to confront them directly.

2 *Ascertain the reason for non-compliance.*

- Side-effects? Explain that these will often slowly decrease and even disappear.
- Unsure of the dosage frequency? Explain, write it out and rehearse it at every review.
- Unable to open the pill bottles? The pharmacist can supply containers with easy-opening caps. But blister packs remain a major problem for many.

- Unable to swallow larger tablets or capsules? This is a common problem. Select smaller presentations or prescribe in liquid formulation.
- Unable to remember the regimen? Simplify the regimen as far as possible, and ask the pharmacist to make up a weekly supply in one of the several good dosage aids – this is especially useful for carers.

3 *Educate at every opportunity*, and ask all your colleagues, GPs, nurses and pharmacists to reinforce the message. Try to do this in the context of a 'therapeutic contract' between the patient and yourself – a 'concordance'. 'We can do together what neither of us can do alone.' It is a part of the process of teaching and conditioning health behaviour.

4 Try giving the patient a *'drug diary'*, to complete daily and bring to you at each review. (This will not suit all patients.)

5 For 'at-risk' patients, *telephonic reminders* have proved very effective, whether by GPs, the nurse, the pharmacist or the reception staff who deal with repeat prescriptions. Many housebound patients welcome this contact with the outside world.

6 At every opportunity, reassure patients that *they will not become addicted to or dependent on their somatic medications* – this is a major worry for many intelligent lay people, which we doctors are not always aware of.

7 Likewise, reassure patients that *the pure drugs you prescribe are much more effective and usually safer than herbal extracts*, which vary greatly in dosage and may contain dangerous impurities such as the plant's own pesticides, which are potentially toxic.

8 *Nationwide media campaigns.* These have proved very effective in predisposing patients to accept their 'therapeutic contract' with the clinician. However, they need to be repeated fairly frequently, as does all advertising, with new formats for each repetition – cartoons, national celebrities, interviews with 'real people', etc. Unfortunately, the Department of Health has not been particularly consistent about this, and campaigns have been 'few and far between'. However, the doctors, nurses and pharmacists in any region could mount short, frequent campaigns in the local media. These can be very effective – there are always a few good media communicators in our ranks who would do this well and enjoy it at the same time! Local newspapers, radio and television are glad to get health inputs with a local 'slant', and at no cost!

The self-medicators: a special subgroup of non-compliant patients

A hundred years ago, the great Canadian physician, Sir William Osler, described humanity as 'the only creature with an intense desire to take medicines!' Humankind has not changed, and the opportunities for self-treating and encouragement to do so are seen in every pharmacy, convenience store and supermarket, not to mention the Internet.

Most people come to no harm in this way, but a small proportion put themselves at serious risk. For example:

1 Patients with any degree of chronic kidney failure may seriously and rapidly worsen their condition by taking aspirin or any NSAID (the author argued at the UK Committee on Safety of Medicines against a General Sales Licence for NSAIDs, but to no avail. These drugs should not be available in non-pharmacy outlets). Further, NSAIDs interact with numerous commonly prescribed drugs.
2 Patients should be warned not to mix herbal remedies with prescription medicines. The *BNF* (Appendix 1) has 19 entries on drug interactions with St John's Wort, and there is a special UK website giving warnings on herbal remedies (www.mhra.gov.uk). Herbal remedies are unstandardised, very impure and most are not subject to the rigorous safety testing of scientific medicines. It is quite wrong to label them 'complementary and alternative medicines', for they should not be used to complement modern drugs, and they are not a comparable alternative to modern drugs except, perhaps, for the 'worried well' who do not need any medicine, but experience a placebo effect which may be satisfying to them.

All primary care clinicians, doctors, pharmacists and nurses should routinely ask patients who are on maintenance medication whether they are taking any such medicines, or indeed sharing a relative's or neighbour's drugs – all of these things happen!

Supplement: some titbits from compliance research

Non-compliance is of two types – intentional and non-intentional. In the first type, the patient makes a decision not to take the medicines, or to take them as and when they choose, and ignore the directions. In the second type, a variety of factors mitigate against the patient's best intentions.

Intentional non-compliance: the patients' perspectives

1 Some believe that their bodies will self-cure, and do not realise that for most chronic diseases that is not the case.
2 Some doubt the efficacy of modern medicines.

3 Some fear that they will become addicted to their drugs.
4 Some believe that their bodies will develop immunity to long-term treatment.
5 Some dislike 'handing over control' of their bodies and/or minds to medicines (and clinicians) – 'loss of autonomy'.
6 Many imagine that a short course of medicine will cure them of hypertension, diabetes, etc.
7 Many do not comprehend the long-term benefits of maintenance medication, or the risks of having no treatment.
8 Some are worried about side-effects, often with good reason.
9 Some fear 'unnatural, synthetic chemicals', preferring 'natural remedies' without realising the risks that herbals may cause.
10 Some have a completely anti-drug attitude, even to the vaccination of their children.

Apart from the last one, all of these reasons for non-compliance have some underlying rationality, from a lay viewpoint, and all are amenable to repeated, reasoned education in an atmosphere of trust and co-operation. In many cases, the outcome of improved well-being will reinforce compliant behaviour. A significant improvement in self-medication in 50% of non-compliant patients would be a reasonable aspiration.

Unintentional non-compliance

Those whose intended compliance with prescribed medication is seriously hindered include:

1 the confused elderly
2 the forgetful and mentally impaired
3 patients on more than three medicines
4 those with poor eyesight (not helped by the small type on pharmacy bottles) and poor literacy
5 those with arthritis of the hand or wrist and those with inadequate co-ordination, trying to open bottles or express tablets from blister packs
6 those who rely on a carer who doesn't understand or follow the medication schedule.

Great improvements can be achieved in all of these patients with a little effort by the professionals, in contrast to the situation with the intentional non-compliers.

References

1 McGavock H, Britten N and Weinman T (1997) *A Review of the Literature on Drug Adherence.* Royal Pharmaceutical Society of Great Britain, London.
2 Cramer JA and Spilker B (1991) *Patient Compliance in Medical Practice and Therapeutic Trials.* Raven Press, New York.

Conclusion

You should now have acquired the basic concepts of how drugs work, at least in sufficient detail to make you a better-informed prescriber and to help you to understand what you are doing when you prescribe. I hope you have enjoyed this topic, which has fascinated me for many years. And a final word of advice – keep the *BNF* in your pocket and refer to it whenever in doubt. If still in doubt, do not prescribe! When you have acquired experience in prescribing, you might wish to develop your knowledge by keeping the companion book, *Pitfalls in Prescribing and How to Avoid Them*, beside your *BNF*.

Hugh McGavock
July 2015

Prescribing safely: a checklist for every prescription

Expert and experienced prescribers usually run the following checklist before issuing every prescription, often as an ingrained habit. It is a very good habit indeed!

1	**Diagnosis:**	how certain is it?
2	**Drug:**	appropriate for the diagnosis? *N.B. avoid NSAIDs unless inflammation is present*
3	**Dose:**	elderly? child? renal failure, liver failure?
4	**Other drugs:**	any interaction? (including OTC and herbals)* *a vital safety check – N.B. NSAIDs*
5	**Route of administration:**	appropriate for clinical situation?
6	**Frequency of dosage:**	agreed and recorded?
7	**Duration of treatment:**	review regularly to determine clinical need
8	**Effective?**	*if not, ask why* – non-compliance? wrong diagnosis? wrong drug? dose too low? enzyme induction? drug interaction?
9	**Side-effects:**	expect them! seek them! report them!

* OTC = 'over the counter', drugs bought without a prescription. Herbal remedies are very impure and unstandardised medicines, given and consumed without adequate diagnosis, follow-up or legal redress for harm caused, e.g. the weakly-effective St John's Wort can lead to oral contraceptive failure.

Index

Entries in **bold** denote tables and boxes; entries in *italics* denote figures.

CPD with Radcliffe

You can now use a selection of our books to achieve CPD (Continuing Professional Development) points through directed reading.

We provide a free online form and downloadable certificate for your appraisal portfolio. Look for the CPD logo and register with us at: www.radcliffehealth.com/cpd

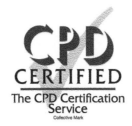